SECRET Truths
Health & Well-Being

HEALTH TRUTHS THAT *EVERYONE* SHOULD KNOW

TOXICITY AND THE NERVOUS SYSTEM

SECRETS BEYOND NUTRITION

Resolve Exhaustion & Tiredness NATURALLY!

Recognise Obstacles to Health and Vitality

Body-Mind and Emotional Impact

MYRA SRI

Energy Healing Secrets Series: 3

COPYRIGHT and LEGAL NOTICE

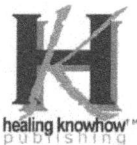

First Published as electronic book in Australia 2015
First printing July 2015
Healing Knowhow™ Publishing,
P.O. Box 126, Toukley, NSW 2263, Australia

healing knowhow™
publishing

National Library of Australia Cataloguing-in-Publication entry:
Sri, Myra, author
Secret truths health & well-being : health truths that
everyone should know, toxicity and the nervous system,
secrets beyond nutrition / Myra Sri.
ISBN: 9780992392437 (paperback)
0992392438
Energy healing secrets series ; 3
Includes bibliographical references
Holistic medicine
Alternative medicine
615.5

Disclaimer

All information provided in this report are based on the author's knowledge, research, experience and personal experiences in the Health, Self-Development, Energy Work and Spiritual fields and are intended to inform, furnish and inspire the reader with options, possibilities, knowledge and natural alternatives.

Any product or supplement recommendations are purely altruistic and there is no personal profit or gain in any other way than passing on the best that the author knows at time of writing.

The Author, Myra Sri, does not intend to make any recommendations or representations that are contrary to common sense or medical supervision. Please consult your health professional if you have any health concerns, and also consider a complementary health-care professional who will further confirm and support your journey to health.

This report is intended to assist the individual toward a more comprehensive understanding with regard to health, energy, self help and self empowerment.

Included:

- What Doctors don't tell you or don't know
- Affirmations to Health
- Suggestions for holistic healing approach

CONTENTS

SECRETS BEYOND NUTRITION...

This book acknowledges the need for proper nutrition and appropriate health care – then goes beyond it! It uncovers some of the hidden truths that prevent us from full recovery and which can compromise our health and vitality. When you think you are doing all the right things, but are still not getting better, this knowledge is BASIC! When the medical profession are scratching their heads and can't pinpoint the problem (or you feel they are sweeping it under the carpet), then this information is a MUST! When you know there is a problem and a reason why you are so tired, yet tests can't find anything wrong, this book is ESSENTIAL!

Some of the issues covered include:

- Well-Being Basics That *Everyone* Should Know
- Hidden Truths Behind Exhaustion and Tiredness
- Body-Mind-Spirit and Emotional Impacts
- Toxicity and the Nervous System
- Dental Amalgams and Mercury
- The Power of Minerals
- Discover Veiled Blockages to Health and Vitality
- Resolve Exhaustion and Tiredness NATURALLY!
- Toxicity Impact on Nervous System, Brain and Body
- Recognise Blocks to Weight-Loss, Health and Brain Function Naturally
- Hidden Personal Power
- Affirmations to Heal and Health
- Positive Energy
- Sensitive Types

BODY, MIND, SPIRIT

Tuesday, 11.50am

Hello.

As a therapist, over the years I have seen a variety of people and often this has meant a variety of issues and ailments.

One thing about self help and natural health and recovery is what the client can do for themself after a session... Giving people further understandings of underlying factors and often providing information for them to be pro-active is important if we are not to become a nation and era of dependent pill-poppers.

Questions get asked about how things got the way they did for the client...what is behind their exhaustion, what are they not doing right, and if they are doing things right then why are these not working for them.

In this book I answer common questions from clients that can be applied whether you are seeing a health professional or not.

You are about to learn of truths other than the obvious reasons for tiredness, exhaustion and depletion of energy from a holistic health professional. Based on client sessions and my own personal experience, I have spent many years working with these issues in a clinical and consultative environment.

There is a growing consensus that we can no longer treat the body and its physical ailments as problems belonging solely to the body and the physical.

And thank goodness that this is now becoming more mainstream as people determine their own health, responsibilities and rights.

Generally, cure does not always last when we simply try to treat the body as a machine. The body may well be magnificent at functioning all by itself for most things, but it can only be pushed for so long before demanding more than customarily being ignored.

More and more people are rediscovering the heart / mind / soul / body connections again after many years, even centuries, of treating these individual components in separation and isolation.

We will be looking at hidden reasons, things that we may well be able to address ourselves or with wise support, that prevent us from gaining full well-being and vitality. Blockages to our recovery and health.

Things we may well have been unaware of before. Things that are unseen contributors and affecters of health and well-being.

We will look at what is required for a healthy body, and some of the major contributors that affect and compromise health for everyone who is unaware of them. This includes the results of impact from the heart and soul on the emotional and mental attitudes toward self healing and expression as well as blockages caused by a variety of sources that limit our health and well-being.

We will also look at common energy systems of the body, as well as the relevant emotional and mental impacts.

Included in this report is a brief look at the Nervous System and Immune System, stubborn weight issues, brain function, positive thinking, meditation and even a quick look at 'spirituality'.

Health is much more than a physical issue, and anyone who has been through a stressful time will recognize that it can take a while to fully recover physically and emotionally back to feeling vital again.

We hope to give you some ideas that we have gathered through digging for personal answers as well as study and practice in the complementary therapies.

SECRET TRUTHS ABOUT HEALTH AND ENERGY

Firstly we cover the health and energy basics, then we will look at the hidden and often secret reasons preventing well-being.

Requirements for Health and Energy

What is required to achieve and maintain a healthy body... your healthy body?

And how does health – or the lack of it - impact on one's life?

To answer these questions it may help if we first take a look at our own current life and decide for our self whether it could be improved upon;

Am I completely happy with the level of energy I have at my command? Am I happy with how I view my life, and my lot in life? Is my appetite normal – normal for myself that is, given my personal energy requirements? Do I feel bloated after I eat? Do I need lots of sugar or other addictive substances to function satisfactorily? Am I asking from my body more than it is capable of giving or willing to give?

It can also be a good exercise to take note of what we find when we take a closer look at the quality of our lives.

Particularly when we look at our body, and the types of energy required to run it.

When we think of energy in relation to the human body, we usually think in the terms of the energy derived from calories. Equating it to the fuel we put in a car. I refer to this as glucose-energy, as this sort of energy is the result of the body breaking down incoming nutrition into useable sugars / glucose which can be utilised easily by the brain and muscles. When everything is functioning correctly, the fuel or calories we take in equals the equivalent output in energy.

This is a general and usual understanding of energy.

Hence we usually think that 'feeling tired', 'exhausted', 'drained', 'done in', 'puffed out' etc is a lack of energy or that it is connected with the quality of our food intake.

If we are eating the correct food, and generally taking reasonable care of ourself, how can we feel exhausted? How can this happen?

Faulty nutrition is the first usual item to address. But if you are eating healthily, then what?

Blockages to health can start with faulty digestion. But there are other factors that create obstacles to well-being for us to look at shortly.

But energy coming from nutrition is not the only source of energy...

However, let us look at issues related to compromised physical energy first.

Problems with Producing Energy

If indeed we are eating in a healthy balanced way yet we are still feeling tired or drained, then we need to look further.

Some common reasons for these symptoms of compromised energy are usually directly related to:

- The body's inability to process, absorb or uptake nutrition correctly
- Incorrect nutrition
- A problem with the body's hydration processes and intracellular integrity
- Immune system overwhelm
- Long term (chronic) stress
- Adrenal exhaustion
- Shock or trauma to the body or person
- Development of 'sensitivities' or worse, allergies
- Overuse of chemicals or substance, whether through prescribed medication or recreational substances
- Lack of appropriate rest, sleep and / or relaxation
- Heavy Metal Toxicity from amalgam fillings & mercury products
- Toxic absorption caused by herbicides, pesticides and certain food additives
- Habitual nightshift work
- Too much or a continued high level of excitement

Any one of the above will interfere with proper digestive functioning. It can also affect the acid balance both in the digestive system and in the body possibly resulting in leaky gut or irritable bowel syndrome, just to name a couple of problems with the digestive system.

13 BASIC HEALTH FACTORS

Food alone does not attain health. There are certain essential factors for the body to thrive and so to deliver its best back to us.

For health and well-being, it is important that the body have the following essential elements or factors of health in order of priority:

1. Air

2. Water

3. Food

4. Sunshine / daylight

5. Sleep / rest

6. Nutrition

7. Exercise

8. Relaxation / fun

9. Personal hygiene

10. Environment

11. Self connection

12. Relationships

13. Emotional, Mental and Spiritual Balance

The first seven items are essential for the body alone to grow, whilst the other elements impact on *how* the body grows and develops. And quality of life.

Some of these basics are obvious, though we can take them for granted.

Water

It is basic commonsense to acknowledge that water is a primary requisite for life after the need for oxygen. We breathe continually, but we tend to drink only when we are thirsty. Those who have been on a detoxification regime or who perform exercise regularly will recognize the need for good quality water and lots of it.

However, due to its increasing importance and relevance in today's world of tendency to contamination from so many sources, here is a word on water. Over the years, the quality of our water has changed. Once we could drink plain tap water with little or no fear of negative consequences.

That being said, copper piping was considered the superior mode of transport to the domestic home. Over time it was discovered that copper piping could affect water if not installed correctly. To those in the know, there is a process that can still render copper as superior. However, domestic plumbers not always being fully informed of this, we turned to plastic. Then we discovered that hot water pipes and hot water cisterns could leach unwanted chemicals into water.

Fast forward to today and we find that domestic treated water has changed a good deal, and with additives of chlorine, and the controversial fluoride being forced onto the population, not to mention other chemical in most states, many have taken to drinking spring or bottled water.

There are arguments for and against bottled water.

Some educated people have upgraded to purified water, and new types of water filtering treatments that can remove the acidic content of water, providing only alkaline water. There are many advancements in reclaiming or creating healthy water that is not necessary to go into here, and some even claim to deliver water similar to 'nature'.

Dr Masaru Emoto has made a study on the types of water structures that support the body and mind and those that don't, and his photographic work on water crystals is very impressive. From an energetic point of view, he has a lot to contribute but also gives us some understanding of how we can enhance our water ourselves.

Coming back to the basics of water, filtering seems to be necessary if not essential. Though the need to filter water so intensively has removed many of the normal bugs that we imbibed along with our friendly H2O and our systems therefore are often no longer so accustomed at dealing with these semi-harmless organisms. Which may present a problem occasionally when it is combined with other substances that the body is having trouble dealing with. But that is not a main concern at this point in this section.

The issue I am attempting to draw attention to is that water, and the quality of that water, is the most necessary and valuable nutrient that our bodies digest via the digestive system. And the integumentary system. The skin and digestion are carriers of fluids not only into the body, but also into the cells, and is required in some form in all functions of our physicality. Air is the number one nutrient, and when this is contaminated it can seriously compromise one's health. Fortunately, we may be able to take steps to remove ourselves from polluted air.

Our water supply, however, is often beyond such control. And we are often dependent on council and government regulations and controls.

Getting the best quality water that you can get, or afford can make a difference to many of the functions in the body. And drinking enough of it is also extremely important.

Many people mistake a 'thirst urge' for water to be a signal to drink something, anything, to satisfy it. Certain fluids do NOT satisfy thirst, and actually only increase the bodies need for more water to process the intake of another laden fluid.

In the elderly, the ability to differentiate thirst from hunger can become dimmed, so there can be confusion and often people will eat something when their body is actually asking for water. If you are not sure which it is, to identify more easily, have a few sips of water first and see if this satisfies the urge.

Can't Swallow

If you are having difficulty drinking enough water, I suggest that you increase your intake. If you find this hard, do what I did when I first started upping my water; Drink at least one or two glasses *before* you have your drink of tea or coffee, then have your hot drink as a reward! If the water is too cold, add a drop of boiled water – this is very beneficial to the stomach and liver. First thing in the morning, add the juice of a lemon into semi-warm water to help to flush the liver.

If you are still having trouble in the swallowing of it, maybe seek the advice and assistance of a kinesiologist or therapist to overcome your 'gag' reflex.

Some people have a resistance to water, and may need a semi-allergic reaction to it dealt with.

My own issue with water meant that I could only swallow it in sips. Until I discovered through a kinesiology session that my body had set up an alert system after a near drowning experience, which had resulted in an automatic constriction of the throat when I had more than a small mouthful to drink.

Once this was cleared together with the associated fear and stress, I could literally guzzle water very easily.

BODY AND ENERGY BASICS - TYPES OF ENERGY

Most of us are aware of certain physical systems in the body, such as the digestive system, the circulation system, the skeletal system, the lymphatic system etc. And some of us have an understanding of the requirements of these systems. This is necessary to support and help heal the physical body, and to maintain its functions. And understanding how our body works is a great start to supporting a healthier and happier life and body.

However, we are more than just our body.

If we were to realize that our body is similar to a house or a hotel even, which accommodates its own staff that run their own independent departments yet they link in with each other for the smooth running of the hotel, so that things happen smoothly, then we may have an idea of how amazingly complicated yet competent the body can be. And of how systems, organs, glands, blood, fluids and electrical messengers (including neurotransmitters, hormones and enzymes) can work together for a flowing and efficient management of the body as a whole. That is *when* it is functioning harmoniously.

Each of these departments require 'goods' from each other in order to continue to function: the stomach requires food to digest, the liver requires processed nutrients from the digestion to revitalize the blood and so feed all departments, the kidneys require fluids and correct minerals to carry electrical impulses to the brain and back to the body (the telephone system if you like), the brain requires sugars (energy) to do its work, the muscles require protein to repair its wear – and so on.

So the body works together without our having to consciously think about what we have to do next. And for most of us, this means that we eat when our stomachs tell us we are hungry and require sustenance, and we drink when our brain is alerted by our kidneys via our mouths that we need more fluids.

Each organ, gland or system requires its own unique nutritional packaging for it to function.

But this is only part of the equation.

Goods arrive, get opened up, unpackaged and processed according to its requirements, then sent to the correct internal destination. That is the basic bit. And handled correctly, it can and will sustain the body for a long time, as long as it is not being abused.

And a hotel can work very well with the correct 'deliveries' of nutritional goods - but what sort of a hotel would it be if one merely showed up for work day in and day out, relentlessly?

There has to be a heart for a hotel, for any residence, for anybody, if one wishes to enjoy the experience and live to the fullest. The heart makes the difference in the *quality* of experience, and helps to lighten the boring and to face the mundane.

To simplify the process of food as nutrition, we are aware that food eventually gets broken down to sugars (energy) and amino-acids (proteins for repair), and this is a whole complicated process which doesn't need to be overly short-circuited by too much refined sugar

As we have seen that is one part of the puzzle.

And there is a lot more to life than just food.

Let us look at the unseen aspects that impact on our health and our energy potential.

Rather than just limiting our perception of physical nutritional energy as being the *only* source of energy in the body, we need to also be aware of some of the other essential energy systems.

These all work together to give a more complete energy picture.

Here is a list of some of the more commonly known energy systems in the body.

- Emotional Energy – Affect of Emotion on The Body / Being

- ElectroMagnetics System - Electrical Balance

- Meridian System – Energy Circuits in the Physical Body

- Chakras – Energy Centers Governing Input and Output of Energy

- The Brain and the Nervous System

Emotion - Affect of Emotion on The Body / Being

Anybody who has ever been sad or even angry can recognize the immediate impact on the body. In sadness there is a drop in energy, a kind of drooping of the body almost, as one processes the emotion. In anger, there is a heating in the body, usually more easily recognized or localized in the head or gut, and there is associated faster breathing and a tendency to body tension or rigidity or readiness for action.

Happiness brings its own reaction, usually accompanied by a lightness in the body, a tendency for the mouth to want to smile, and a release of easy flowing energy.

So emotion impacts on the body. For both men and women.

The following is just my general observations and is not a condemnation or judgment, but rather a highlighting of how the genders tend to handle emotional issues. For from my perspective I have noted that there is a difference in the way men and women handle and respond to emotion. I say this with the understanding of a need and natural tendency for each sex to have some aspect of the other sex as part of them – that both men and women have within them the seeds of the other. What I mean by this is that within men there is often a hidden softer female side, though it can be buried deep, yet give them a favourite dog or a new baby to hold and you will see it emerge.

And within women there is often a buried male side, and this tends to come out when they decide to stand up to a bully or when they dare to seize hold of a career opportunity. And the degree of male to female balance within each of us can be quite individual and emerge differently over different issues depending on our predispositions. So let's look at what each of these aspects or sides of us does when it comes to the emotions... Though I talk of men and women, I am indicating the general female attitude toward emotion and the general male attitude toward emotion and their differences.

Day to day, women tend to be more readily affected by emotion than men – again this is a general remark and indicative of the female response to it, as there are some men who are in tune with their emotions or who respond quickly to intense emotion. However, women generally do tend to feel or acknowledge or react to emotion quicker.

Again let me say that this is not a criticism at all, just a general observation, for where would we be without the quick responses from caring women? However, it appears to me that both men and women have lessons regarding handling emotions.

Even just the list of emotions experience by the sexes tends to give a clue – men recognize fear, joy, anger, sadness, despair, elation. Women's emotional vocabulary will allow them to recognize the degrees and nuances in emotion – exhilaration, exquisiteness, heartsick, despondent, dubious, charmed, vulnerable, concerned, blissful, tentative, decimated, anguish, bothered, affectionate etc – the list is pretty big...

For men there tends to be an equating of emotion with a lack of control. And a lack of reason or logic. Usually men don't like it (the emotion, often *any* emotion) and try to control it, often putting it in a box to be sorted later - or never – as they never quite trust emotion. So they try to ignore it, or they fear it. Until it accumulates and sneaks up on them and then they may well explode or collapse. Acknowledging an emotion and addressing it is a mature lesson for men.

Whilst women have a different problem. For them, they are generally brought up to explore or express their emotion rather than repress it as men are often taught. When women go into their emotion, they may find it hard to find their logical side in this, and the emotion can take over, causing them to have to swim in it. And sometimes drown in it. For managing so many emotions that they can acknowledged somewhere within their being can be a trial. Rising above the emotion and putting on the 'logical' hat to reason their emotion is a mature and often hard-earned skill for women.

And interestingly, each sex can learn from the other just how to do what they need to do to be comfortable around emotion – in order to MANAGE it, for that is the lesson they are both learning.

It would also appear that women generally genetically tend to be more geared to quick emotional response in this way in order to respond to the needs of any offspring. Just as a man is geared to overcome his emotions to get on with the job of protection and guardianship. Neither is wrong, just different emotional and energetic approaches and handling of emotion.

Within each sex or gender, there are also those who are the more sensitive, not just to sensation or excitement, but also to emotion.

And I am sure that each of us has seen someone at some time ruled strongly by powerful emotion and unable to think straight. Just as we have seen someone so logically headstrong that they ignore all normal emotional response or acknowledgement. Emotion exists and is a part of human life.

It can be like some sort of frequency being broadcast in the air, and someone has to act like the radio receiver to act on it and so move it along and out of the way...

Interestingly if for whatever reason, a man or a woman is in denial of a strong emotion, it may fall to a child or a more sensitive person in the immediate family or vicinity to feel or sense that emotion.

Rather than us getting caught up on who is or should be feeling what, let us just say that generally the most sensitive will 'feel' any strong emotion in a family situation, and will often try to process it. This may mean that they will possibly perceive the strong emotion as something that they are responsible for, or will try to fix it, or hide it or any number of things. Sometimes, they will play up, and will be perceived as a 'problem'. Let me be clear that this is not necessarily the absolute or only rule with a 'problem' child, but can be the more common reason.

Emotion then, is something that can have a strong effect even though we cannot see it or touch it.

We may possibly regard emotion as something strong that overtakes us, and we have no say in the matter. The truth about emotion is that it is actually just energy.

Yes, that's right – it is just energy.

> ## *Emotion = E-motion*
> ## *E-Motion = <u>E</u>nergy in <u>Motion</u>*

Nothing in life is static, everything is in a process of change, and there are so many reasons for energy to be moving in life that we cannot possibly cover them all here. But when we have energy moving and emerging as an emotion, then we are challenged to deal with it.

So what is emotion?

Put simply, it is an energy flowing through the body that has been labeled with a particular emotion by the 'feeler' in order for them to identify it and deal with it. Some call it life-force, as if this energy flow were to stop, we would have no impulse to be inspired, motivated, caring, sympathetic, compassionate, ambitious or passionate about anything.

We learn what to label an emotion because we associate the feeling with the label we hear others putting on it. How did you learn to call that hot intense feeling you felt when someone outraged you by taking your ice-cream away or throwing your toy into the bin or whatever else it was that got you so riled up and you wanted to do something about it?

You probably learned it through your parents, who told you not to get so angry about it, and who possibly insisted

30

that you hide the emotion away so they didn't have to deal with it. We struggle with the feeling and we hear it called something and that's how we remember it. And not to let it cause the dissatisfaction or disapproval (or threat) that we saw on our caregivers face.

What often happens growing up is that we also become scared of the intensity of a strong emotion, and often have not been privy to seeing strong emotion managed in a positive, beneficial or successful way by the mature ones around us, so we get scared of it. We often see our parents or caretakers struggling with strong emotion, especially anger, so we avoid it.

The problem with anger is that we can bury it, push it down and try and reason it out, but it will build up like a volcano, and seek temporary 'pressure' release every so often, usually with or through a totally unrelated event. This is what can happen with unmanaged emotion.

So much of this can be stored in the body. Unknowingly. And for a long time...

Energy and Emotion

Science is now navigating the various pathways of particular perceptions of emotions and the resulting hormonal, neurological and neural effects on the functions of the body.

Emotion affect hormones, hormones produce mood and precursors to emotions. So we can create a kind of cycle of states of feelings and reactions if we do not address breaking or attending to the cycle.

Hormones are responsible for every single activity in the body, and are not just the domain of women. It is now becoming more readily recognised that not only women, but even men suffer from a hormonal crisis in mid-life, as things change in the way the body and brain functions.

So why can this create tiredness in the human body?

Well, battling to batten down our anger, pain or sadness takes a lot of effort.

We may put on a brave face, but eventually we no longer have the free energy to do this, as we exhaust our nervous system in the constant fight to control it. It may take years, but eventually something 'gives' and this often leads to depression. Or other symptoms like Chronic Fatigue, allergies and sensitivities, a weakened Immune System or other disease in the body.

This is not necessarily consciously recognised, as often we have become accustomed to something not being 'quite right' and have learned to navigate and manage our lives around these upsets. Rather than be reminded of them we generally try to forget them as quickly as possible.

Particularly if there appears to be nothing that we can do about them. Such as past abuse, betrayal or rejection.

Consciously we can learn to get past it, but sub-consciously we often make certain decisions about life in order to avoid the same pain or fear or fear of the pain again. Some things can be so buried in our past that we cannot even remember them.

But the body does. The nervous system does.

The subconscious does. And it is ever vigilant to protect us from the same thing happening again.

This can compromise our adrenal system, and also create a 'hair-trigger' reaction in the brain, usually in the amygdala and cerebellum at the brain stem, in relation to anything connected with this past event.

The body does an amazing job to protect us. And this is often one of those things that we are not even aware of.

Most sensitivities are the body's way of saying 'I remember that ... (substance, person, place, judgment etc)...and it caused me to feel (or was present when I felt) ... significant pain / embarrassment / fear / loss / shock etc. Watch out, it could happen again!'

This is how we learn to avoid danger repeating itself.

You can prove this yourself if you have ever had an accident in a place that you are familiar with.

I once had an accident when a car came out from a side street at an intersection that I traveled daily for years. It was a red car, and sure made a mess of mine.

Even though the accident happened on just one day after a 5 year period of daily travel, *every single time* I passed that intersection again *afterwards*, I ALWAYS remembered the accident!

And the red car!

This is one of the body and brain's ways of protecting us.

Unresolved psychological or emotional trauma can be stored away, creating an unseen stress condition which can adversely affect the endocrine system (and hormones). This may well set health problems in motion which may not show up for years.

60% of the general population has psychological stress which includes a very high percentage of chronic illness.

Any kind of trauma is also registered and remembered in the body until dealt with at some later stage.

We currently live in a society that generally seems to believe that if you are no longer under stress, then you should be functioning exactly as immediately before the stress – and without any after effects!

Ridiculous!

Electromagnetics System - Electrical Balance

The human body has its own electromagnetic field (EMF), similar to that of the Earth.

It usually gets bathed in the Earth EMF at night time, helping reset and rejuvenate the external electrical aspects of the human body.

Referred to as the Schumann Resonances, these Earth EMF's are essential for night rest, for the sun and its solar rays are at rest from its daily impacts, and the body now has time to deal with the day's intake, impacts and events whilst processing, repairing and resting from daily activity.

Correct EMF tone and support assists the Immune System. Electro-pollution may cause us to feel more stressed, fatigued and "out of balance." It is now clear through laboratory research that exposing living cells to the a frequency known as the Schumann Resonance had the effect of "protecting" them from ambient and local EMF's, allowing the cells to increase their immune protection, and decrease the absorption of depression-inducing chemicals.

The Schuman Resonance is identified and associated with the natural electrical impulses and frequencies of the planet in natural settings.

Some researchers believe that by producing a 7.83 Hz pulse with a field generator (using a Schumann device); we can counter the effects of these irritating man-made fields that impact on our electrical systems and our electromagnetic fields. By replicating the Earth's natural rhythm, we may be providing ourselves (at least in our immediate vicinity) with a healthier environment.

Getting away from electro pollutants as much as possible will help the body reset and feel more relaxed or 'lighter'.

Too much electrical machinery or being too close to a lot of electrical appliances, or sleeping by electrical circuit boards will certainly compromise our EMF and affect our quality of rest and restoration.

Finding ways to better support our nervous system, our energy systems, our electromagnetic field and all of those unseen communication signals that take place within the body will obviously enhance our health and well-being. Discovering those things, or at the very least, being more aware of the possibilities of those things that can compromise our health will allow us to make better choices as well as to take charge of our healing process.

If the Immune System is toned and functioning correctly, we can resist any number of potential physical problems. Indeed, a healthy immune system is a major key to optimal health.

If our electromagnetic system is functioning properly, we not only have better physical function in the body, we also have healthier energy fields which can often be communication systems in themselves.

It may well be worth noting here that electronic and electrical devices are not the only things that can affect our own EMF. Humans themselves can have a unique frequency of their own in their EMF that can be changed according to emotion, state, agitation or a number of other things.

We can reclaim a more natural flow in our energy systems when we are in harmony with the natural rhythm of the planet, or within our self. Obviously meditation can help some people, nature can assist others, art and music can support still others and there are many ways that we can rebalance our own energies and our own EMF.

When we are in flow, we have less chance of affecting another negatively, too.

This can also alert us to the possibility that when we are around aggravation frequencies put out by others, this can impact on our own energy capabilities. What one can do about such things is covered further in *"Secrets Behind Energy Fields"* however the following may explain what you can experience when being around certain others.

Personal Frequency Electromagnetics

To understand more clearly about our personal energy systems and how they can be impacted by external forces, let us look at a simplified model of energy frequencies.

Our energy systems are imbued with electromagnetic qualities: this means that they possess both transmitting – electro or electric – and magnetic – attracting abilities. This means that our energy systems not only senses energies or incoming frequencies, but also sends out energies or vibrationary frequencies.

To demonstrate simply how the energy anatomy can interact with another's energy anatomy, the following illustrations show a simplified radiating frequency. For our purpose, we are only looking at the general overall energy surrounding the body, including the electromagnetic attributes which includes the energy output and the energy input or impact.

The first illustration attempts a sense of one persons personal wave pattern frequencies – let's call this person A – when they are in personal harmony or balance.

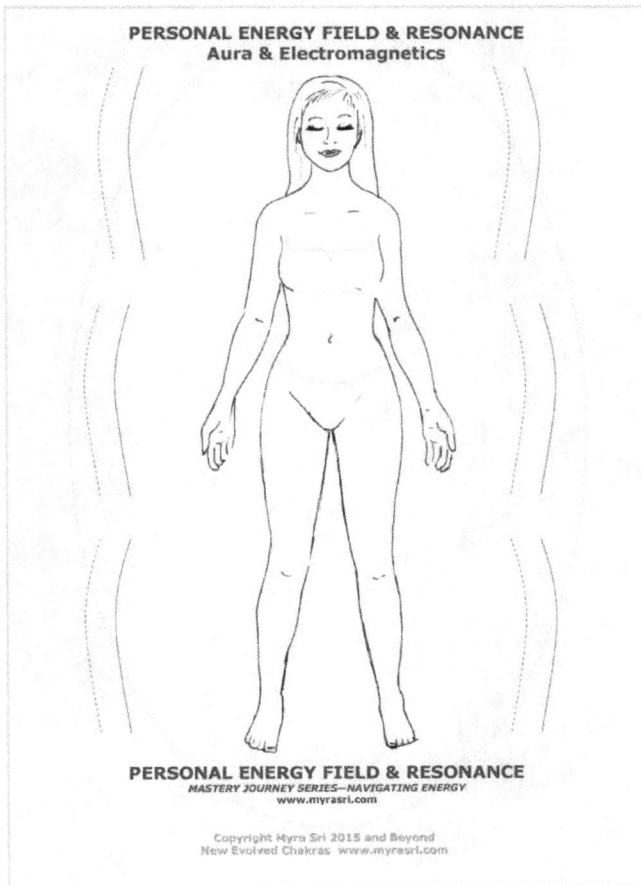

PERSONAL ENERGY FIELD & RESONANCE
Aura & Electromagnetics

PERSONAL ENERGY FIELD & RESONANCE
MASTERY JOURNEY SERIES—NAVIGATING ENERGY
www.myrasri.com

Copyright Myra Sri 2015 and Beyond
New Evolved Chakras www.myrasri.com

Now let's introduce another person (B) and their energy systems into the equation. This person's frequency is also generally in personal balance.

If their frequency contains similar resonances and vibrations we may well have harmony.

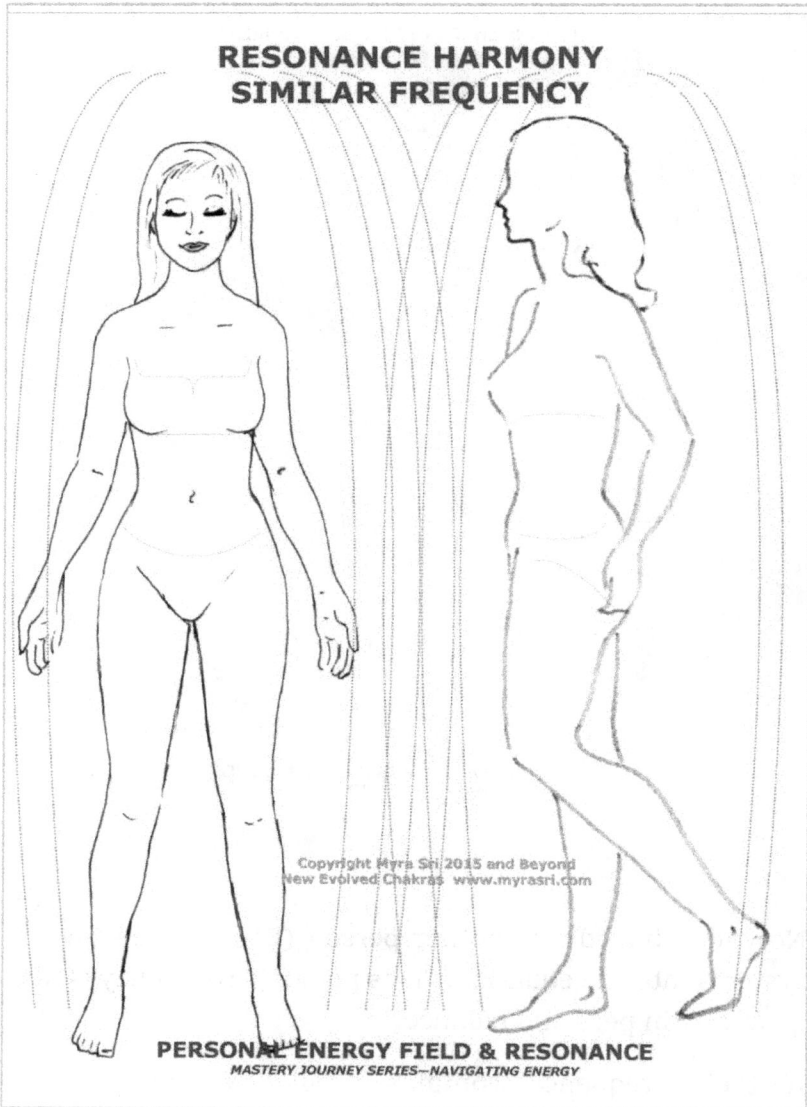

**RESONANCE HARMONY
SIMILAR FREQUENCY**

Copyright Myra Sri 2015 and Beyond
New Evolved Chakras www.myrasri.com

PERSONAL ENERGY FIELD & RESONANCE
MASTERY JOURNEY SERIES—NAVIGATING ENERGY

So far, so good.

The similarities in frequencies does not create any apparent disturbances.

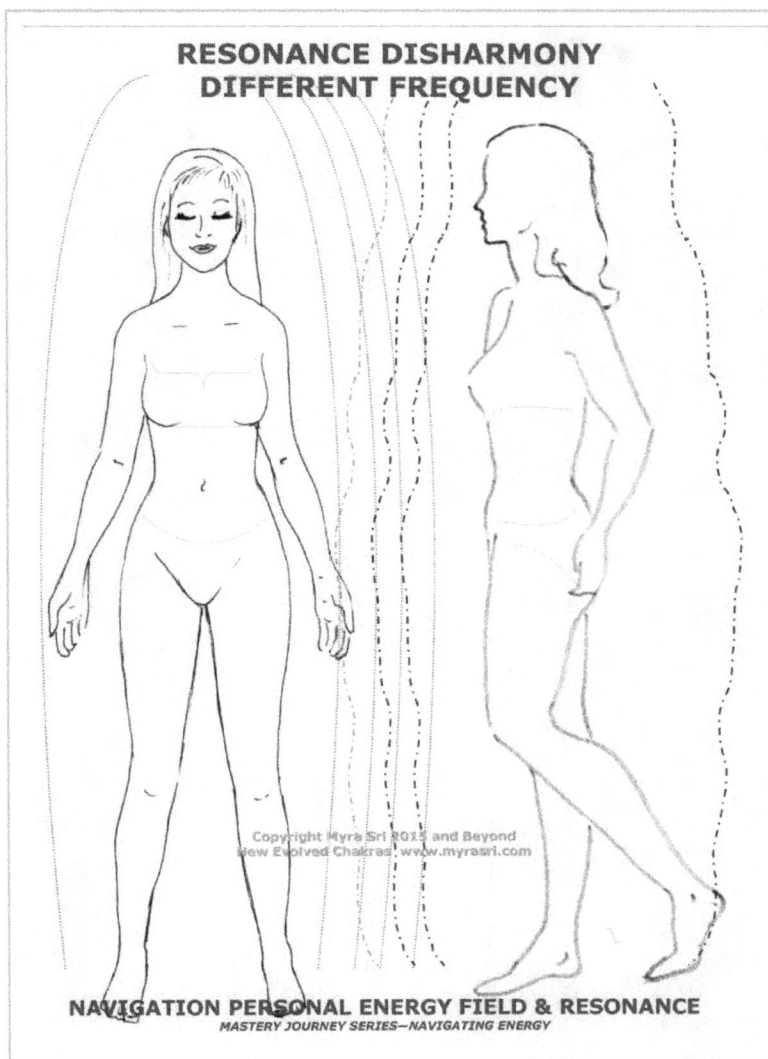

**RESONANCE DISHARMONY
DIFFERENT FREQUENCY**

Copyright Myra Sri 2015 and Beyond
New Evolved Chakras, www.myrasri.com

NAVIGATION PERSONAL ENERGY FIELD & RESONANCE
MASTERY JOURNEY SERIES—NAVIGATING ENERGY

However, when another's energy field vibrations and therefore their EMF field carries a different frequency, it may possibly affect one's own field. Compare this in the next illustration.

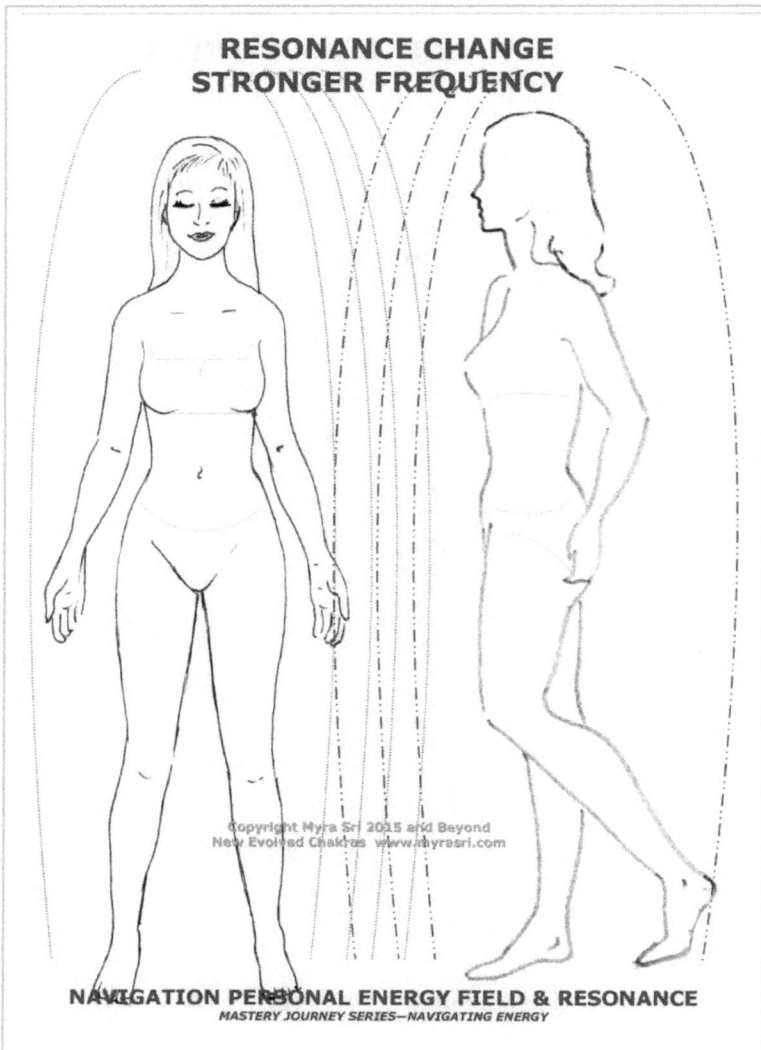

RESONANCE CHANGE
STRONGER FREQUENCY

NAVIGATION PERSONAL ENERGY FIELD & RESONANCE
MASTERY JOURNEY SERIES—NAVIGATING ENERGY

If someone else's field (B) is highly charged or more intensely powered, however temporary, it can impact and sometimes overwhelm or override another's (A) energy systems via the EMF.

What Does This Mean?

This of course can depend on the tone, strength or vibrancy of the "receiving" energy field (A's). If the tone is good, there is less likelihood of overwhelm etc, or at least, there is some warning or sensory perception of the "invasion".

In the final image, there may be a transmission or simply a sense of irritation or aggravation for example, from (B) or a sense of unsettling-ness. If the difference in frequency is due to some negative emotion, memory or experience, sometimes it can actually create a similar vibration or resonance in A. This can then translate into a sense of irritation or disruption within A's energy systems of functions. On occasion, the very issues or symptoms that have been introduced by the disharmony of B can be played out in the experiences of A.

Sometimes the difference in frequency has nothing to do with what each is going through, simply that there is a possibly basic incompatibility of energy. No matter how good things are for each person individually, they may never be able to fully relax around each other simply because of the difference/s.

All of the above energy and electrical energy interchanges and interactions or impact depends on the state of the two energy fields or EMF's involved.

This is a very simplified explanation, but it can give a visual clue as to not only how energy fields are impacted, which will relate to human conditions and energy communication but also, to a degree, on how electronic devices can impact the human EMF.

Nervous System and Chakras – Energy Centers Governing Input and Output of Energy

Most people have heard of the word 'chakras' somewhere, whether through TV or some celebrity associated with spirituality or eastern religion. The word simply means 'wheel', describing the unseen wheels of light and energy that form them.

These energy centres are not necessarily visible to the naked eye, although those with clairvoyant sight and those sensitive to energy can see or feel them. Chakras look a bit like wheels and are spinning vortices of colour and light.

When looking at the physical body, it is interesting to note that where there is the claim that a chakra is placed there, it physically correlates with a large group of ganglionic nerves, congregated together. These nerves lead into the nervous system, and the brain.

So you can choose to look at the attributes solely of the nervous system, or of the chakra system, or even combine them together. For in the eastern traditions, these centers of energy (chakras) both receive messages or information, and transmit them.

I think it safe to say that the receiving of messages is certainly connected with the nervous system. Just thinking of a time when you were in sympathy with someone and felt what they felt will confirm this.

So what about the transmitting of messages or information?

We already know about the different types of nervous systems - the autonomic, the sympathetic and the central. Well, I have certainly felt messages coming from others when standing near them – mostly warm, pleasant and loving. Though I do remember picking up nasty or prickly feelings or messages in the form of projected feelings coming from others that were not friendly toward me or another person. And I have even felt sick when someone projected their energy toward me in a malevolent way.

So for me, I do get this correlation.

These centers, whether you choose to think of them as part of the nervous system or the chakra system, gather and interpret information.

In his book *"Acupuncture and the Chakra Energy System"* (page 55), John R Cross states that his experience working with patients using TCM led him to believe that the energy flow of some meridian energies equated to the flow of the cerebro-spinal fluid.

He noted the links between the body organs and the meridian energy flows, but stated that he has been attempting to figure out whether the links are energetic, reflected, triggered or nervous system. And his conclusion is that it matters not.

I tend to agree and think each has the capacity to affect the other.

Chakras can register incoming energy, both positive and negative.

Sometimes a shock or trauma will affect you in a way that you feel like you have been punched in the stomach or even in the head.

We may not always understand exactly what message is being sent, but this energetic transmitting and receiving of energy certainly makes itself known in the physical body, even though there has been no physical contact, touch or tangible attack.

Prevention is Better Than Cure

Whether you talk about chakras or nervous system issues, the point is that these are related to energy flows, and when these are blocked or backed-up in any way, it creates problems in the body and energy function.

Western medicine can trace when it has become 'solidified' in the physical body, but dealing with it energetically first may well go a long way to reducing, if not eliminating, the problem.

The Brain and the Nervous System

Having outlined the Nervous System connections with the chakra system above, let us take a look at the brain.

This amazing mass of soft tissue is responsible for so many functions in the body, and so very capable of repair and redirection when given the right nutrition, support and encouragement. It is a kind of co-ordination and control centre for many bodily functions and thought processes. Though interestingly it does not contain the whole of the mind of a person. But that is another story.

The brain is linked to the nervous system which travels from the base of the spine up into the brain stem and into the brain. It is one of the first things that forms in early development after conception.

Several medical and neurological models use a three brain system: basically they are the early reptilian brain system of basic instinctive survival reactions, the corpus collosum (mammalian) mid-brain (emotional and social processing) and the cerebral cortex or higher brain (for reasoning).

Besides this model the brain has often been referred to as a "split-brain" system, referring to the apparent separation of left and right hemispheres of the brain, responsible for different brain functions – left brain for detail, analysis, time, step by- step, and the right brain for creativity, bigger picture ability, spatial awareness, and imagination.

Both of these models, the three-brain and the split-brain system, have been further researched and updated and we now have clearer understandings of how they work.

The brain tends to use a network of neurotransmitters, which connect with little electrical charges and over time, repeated experiences or actions can cause a kind of highway of neural links. This allows for us to learn something and to later perform it without having to think about it again – such as driving a car. Step by step at first, until we can zoom along from A to B and be so automatic with our driving that we sometimes cannot even remember how we arrived at our destination. But this can also kind of wire us in to bad experiences too. And shock can overwhelm us electrically so that we can kind of blow a fuse and find that our body or our brain momentarily loses its usual way of being.

When we get 'stuck' or short-circuited in this wiring of the neurotransmitters of one or the other parts of the brain, it can complicate life. Whatever model we use, the brain can get 'saturated' when it has been under long-term emotional stress or stuck when it has been in survival mode for too long, like a record that has become fixed in a groove and can't jump out onto another track.

Depression is a typical result of this sort of long term experience.

Getting both sides of the split-brain to communicate gives us many more options, as does freeing up our brain system from being stuck in the lower brain 'survival' mode or the purely reasoning centre (or even in between). When we gain access to all aspects of the brain energetically and neurologically, our options become more real, practicable and comprehensive.

So what can cause this lack of communication or integration in the brains neural network system?

48

Several things, besides the basics of lack of good quality air, food and water:

Lack of Brain Hydration – the body and in particular the brain, needs not just water but electrolytes (multi-minerals can assist) in water for proper electrical conduction to aid electrical messages between brain and body. Besides water, Magnesium is a key hydrator

Shock – a significant emotional shock can 'freeze' the body or brain, or overwhelm the tissues with huge outputs of adrenaline, aldosterone or cortisol, which can create toxicity. Long term stress through shock will saturate body and brain with toxins released from a system unable to deal with or solve the dilemma

Faulty nutrition – a diet of high fats and low lipids will clog the brain. Fish oils and the omega oils help support the brain, and may assist in staving off brain and memory aging

Faulty digestion – a system that is not properly breaking down its nutrition because of lack of enzymes, over-acidity, irritable bowel, or other gastric problems will not be able to provide the brain with the energy it requires and the brain will 'starve'

Poor circulation – the body usually gives first preference to supply the torso with rich blood, and then the rest of the body. It considers the head as an extremity, like the arms and legs. If your feet and hands are often cold, do check your circulation, as your brain may also be suffering!

Substance abuse – alcohol will literally 'pickle' the brain, as well as wilt healthy neurotransmitters. If you want to avoid thinking, then this will work, but you also risk your limbs and organs being unable to function as before, and some are finding motion impairment a heavy price for their continual partying. Social drugs, though sometimes mimicking a 'spiritual' experience will cloud the brain and energy fields and even damage them

Toxic Overload – substances that we are unaware of such as mercury toxicity in tooth amalgam fillings that poison the brain and body. More on mercury later

Trauma by violence – continual subjection to violence for a period of time will lock the brain into what some call 'stupid' mode. The brain will not be able to see any other reality than the violence it knows. It will not be able to think of other possibilities, and will view life from a narrow perception based on the experiences received. This takes a lot of time and patience, as well as wisdom, love and willingness to heal, to sort out. After the war, there were a lot of 'shell shocked' people that only time out in total peace and support eventually helped.

For the brain to be reintegrated and nourished back to health again try these: Counselling, correct nutrition, chiropractic, Neuro Linguistic modalities, Kinesiology, Brain Hydration formats (kinesiology), Homeopathy, TCM – particularly the herbs, acupuncture, massage, exercise, nature, Feldenkrais a form of body work – very gentle but profound.), NET and Cranio-Sacral Technique all help toward this end.

In particular, address hormonal imbalances such as an overwhelm of cortisol, adrenal hormone overload, dopamine, a lack of serotonin and other 'happy hormones', using the above therapies and nutritional support. It also helps to find something you enjoy and do it, whether it is some doodling or artwork, creating something, learning to cook or enjoying a good book or three.

Nutritional support, or Chinese Herbal medicine can assist some. Massage can release and essential oils can support etherically.

Other supports that may assist are Tai Chi, Qi Gong, Yoga, Core strengthening work.

The Immune System

The Immune System is our first line of defense. Like the Skin, it protects us. It is like a boundary line on the inner level.

It deals with invading toxins and bacteria, and the disposal of unwanted, used up and discarded waste products, carrying them from the body to leave clear pathways for energy and nutrition.

Don't allow negative stuff to accumulate, in your body, or in your life.

In your mind, or in your heart.

The Immune System

A compromised Immune System will not allow the body to heal quickly.
On a metaphysical level, the immune system is about our defences and our self protection. If we don't feel safe or protected, or if we feel that our defences are limited or that we are under attack, this will often affect our immune system.
If we don't have peace within, this will also weaken our immune system.
Seek peace.
Work on your inner strength and security.

By the same token, don't focus on 'them' being 'out' to get you. Change jobs, or environment, or whatever. Deal with your personal relationships, get rid of 'victim' mentality, look for your own choices in situations.

Do what you have to do to gain more peace in your life.

These things *will* strengthen your Immune System.

Adrenal Exhaustion

One little known reason for tiredness is after one has experienced extended periods of stress, or undergone trauma that hasn't yet been completely dealt with or healed. Abuse victims can experience this, and the symptoms are similar to those diagnosed as Post Traumatic Stress Disorder (PTSD).

The adrenals are tiny little glands that sit on the kidneys and provide the adrenaline that spurs us into action. Continual adrenaline action can compromise their function and a long enough period of quality recovery is usually enough to rebalance and recharge them correctly after their effort. The adrenaline can also build up in the body, causing a toxic situation.

Some time ago I came face to face with my own experience of adrenal exhaustion.

I was still working as a therapist at the time, but using the same health and healing tools on myself was not getting the same positive results for me that I was able to achieve with my clients and friends.

Something was obviously wrong.

Well, the fact is that back then my main issue of tiredness and an unusual though associated weight gain was viewed as a thyroid-weight related problem by natural therapists; though normal doctors couldn't diagnose this properly. Because I had reasonable blood pressure and seemed ok in other areas that they could measure, the medical profession didn't think any further action was necessary.

I then had thyroid tests done by a complementary health doctor and we discovered that there *was* a thyroid problem which correct nutritional supplementation and support helped. Now the thyroid hormones were showing ok, but the problem of exhaustion and weight gain still continued. I was showing hair loss, puffiness, depression and a few more other uncomfortable symptoms. This doctor could see that I was eating and doing all the right things yet still suffering.

Moving onto testing for the Reverse T3 hormone function showed a different story to us and confirmed that this hormone was indeed out of whack, as well as my cortisol levels (a by-product of adrenaline), which were, to put it bluntly, ridiculous!

You may need to know that some of the background to all of this had been a recent trauma I had experienced that had triggered other previous traumas that the body (and my heart I guess) had buried in the effort to get on with life. I had had more than most people's share of tragedy and abuse, which had taken its toll in and on my body, though I had valiantly carried on – probably because I hadn't actually known how to do it any differently at the time!

Long term stress will compromise the normal function of the adrenals and can create a continual 'alert' state which eventually wears these important glands out, or exhaust them. A bit like the starting motor in a car getting kind of stuck and being continually turned over even whilst you are driving – wears out the motor (and battery) in the end.

I had a history of a series of stresses without having had the support or safe space to fix them and recharge.

I found that I had weight gain issues and the associated puffiness and exhaustion were simply symptoms of what had gone before, and also the body's way of letting me know it simply couldn't cope nor carry on as before.

Now, this complementary health doctor uncovered the Reverse T3 problem together with the cortisol overload and a leptin-resistance problem, and after working with her treatments, I started to regain my health again. After a year of this treatment, I was called overseas (again) to help out with some family issues (again). This was quite exhausting too, and when I returned back to my home country I was of course now living in a different place so could no longer access this original doctor.

Then more family issues – a family member stealing all of our parents money from them and attempting to abuse then even when they had been admitted to a nursing home took me overseas again, to attempt to sort it out with other family members for my mum and dad together. Because the church protected this person's actions (she was and still is a supposed Christian Minister), she got away with it, so after doing what I could for family, I arrived back and I tried to pick up where I had left off.

Lack of funds saw me visiting the local doctors for support instead at that time.

I was exhausted again.

But the normal medical doctors couldn't diagnose it, insisting that I do Thyroid tests first, and that if these showed a problem, *only* then would they do adrenal tests to see if there was any problem. And of course, because I had worked on my thyroid issues, these showed fine.

Going back for these results was interesting. Even though I was insisting on still having adrenal tests, the doctor simply and point-blank *refused* to do anything about them because my thyroid tests showed ok (no Reverse T3 test was considered either of course).

When I asked him then to account for why I was feeling like I was, he had absolutely *no* answer and still refused me an adrenal test! 'We can't find anything wrong' was his response.

He actually was not interested in helping me, probably labeling me negatively in some way. And I realized that by his actions he was showing disbelief in my symptoms! And in me!

Not long after, I suffered Severe Depression and was forced to take anti-depressants. With a different doctor, thank you. I was actually quite ready to end it all by then, and simply could not stop crying at the drop of a hat. I had sworn never to use anything like this, but realized that I could not cope with life at that point without taking this dreaded medication.

So for a period of eight months I took these pills which controlled the symptoms, but at the same time I was working intensively with an energy healer and kinesiologist to clear out my old stresses. This gave me some equilibrium, and I took myself off the anti-depressants as soon as I could do so safely.

At the same time, I was seeing Traditional Chinese Medicine practitioners, to help me with the tiredness and the terrible cold sweats I was experiencing, whether I was hot or cold.

I was to come to realize that my adrenals were so badly exhausted that they had affected my kidney function. The adrenals sit on top of the kidneys like little hats, and they are closely connected and can even share the load together. I would sweat when I felt a bit cold and then I would feel any breeze rip through my skin like shafts of ice.

Clothing would get wet, I would lose essential minerals through my sweating, and I would get a wet panel from the top of my head down my back past my waste to my hips. I just couldn't get warm... I would need to change clothes three or so times a day, and took to wearing mostly tee-shirts (*tres attractif!*). Putting on more clothes, scarves, jumpers etc only caused me to sweat more. Argh!

Apparently mine was an extreme case, but it also classically demonstrated what happens when the kidney energy, 'chi' as it is called, is compromised. Using further TCM-speak, it was also plain that my Triple Warmer / Burner which simply means, metabolism, digestion, circulation, hormones and a whole lot of other functions in the body, was quite out of whack, and as one TCM practitioner said, 'your thermostat is broken'.

My body was having difficulty in regulating temperature, energy, fluid balance and other functions.

Hot days were no better, and I would freeze in 35° Celsius too, and yet still piling on clothes to stop the breezes from making me feel like I was freezing again.

I found that going out at all was becoming a real challenge.

Discovering what the problems were was a *great* help, and using Chinese prescribed herbs and acupuncture, I began to improve again. They worked on nourishing the kidneys and adrenals as well as my Triple Warmer. And I just kept energetically working on the underlying past stresses and traumas that had contributed.

It didn't happen overnight, but it did eventually happen.

So working on the adrenals and kidneys began to reduce the sweating. And slowly energy began to return.

There were still some other issues to sort out, but the reduction in these horrible temperature shifts was a major relief. Monitoring my stress levels and making sure I took time out to just relax and 'be' also began to help me, and as I had moved closer to the bay, this, for me, was also a part of my healing.

There are some wonderful nutritional supports for helping the adrenals, though I would recommend one focuses on nourishing, rather than activating the adrenals. When they have repaired and rebuilt themselves, then one can start to 'push' them again.

The things that worked well for me included Siberian Ginseng, which is an adaptogen – helps the body in stressful situations. It can also nourish the adrenals. Another remedy is Rhodiola. Also check your iron levels.

And be kind to yourself!

Adrenal Lessons

What I learned about adrenal exhaustion was this:

- Normal medicos are hard pressed to accurately diagnose it
- Most of them don't think in those terms anyway
- Chronic stress or acute stress can trigger it
- It can be behind or allied to PTSD and Depression
- TCM can help, or a good nutritional doctor
- Best to use an energy healer at the same time
- Cortisol is a poison in the body long term, so healthy diet is important for recovery
- Take care with herbs, don't push the adrenals or kidneys too hard to fix, but focus on nourishment
- Plenty of water, fresh foods, nature and some creativity where possible
- Avoid stressful movies, video games, dramatic people, arguments, stressful situations which only re-engage you and perpetuate the condition
- When you begin to recover and fill your 'batteries' of energy again, *do not* go and give it away again (by doing a good deed, or something for someone else). Hold the 'I feel good for now' feeling to yourself; if you share it straight away, you will have a flat battery and feel flat very quickly
- Put yourself first before everyone else or you may find it very hard to recover

OTHER OBSTACLES TO HEALTH AND HEALING

In this section:

Body

- **Inflammation**

- **Mercury Toxicity**

- **Minerals and Vitamins**

- **Excess Weight**

Mind and Spirit

- **Psychological Blocks**

- **Reasons Not to Change**

- **Positive Thinking**

- **Spirituality**

- **Sensitives**

- **Affirmations to Health**

Let us explore more reasons for tiredness and poor health.

We are far more than just our bodies, and we are not just our emotions. (Emotion – e-motion – energy in motion; motion therefore means that the emotion will – eventually - pass.)

We are also not just the sum total of our thoughts. Nor are we just our energy bodies. Yes, these are all part of us, but we are much more than these.

We often try to avoid pain, and indeed, why not? But a certain amount of pain needs to be accepted – to a degree

– as part of life. Pain in the body is actually a warning sign of blocked energy, and that the body (or ourself) needs attention.

Our body will at first whisper to us. If we choose to ignore it, then it will raise its voice.

Often some only listen when the body is literally shouting at them. By this time we often just want to shut it up, so we reach for the quick fix, the magic tablet. What we may not realise is that by this time, byt the time the body is shouting out loud for attention it is often now more complicated than it was, and if we do not pay proper attention, then we may just be dealing with the symptoms and not the real cause.

The fact that a river has dried up, and no longer flows does not necessarily mean that there is no more water – it may possibly mean that a dam has formed, or that it has been siphoned off elsewhere.

Energetic dams whether trauma, accumulated stress, buried emotion, toxicity or whatever, need to be cleared, and the drains cleared and sealed for the flow to begin again.

Inflammation

Inflammation is fast being acknowledged as a major culprit of pain in the body.

With the proliferation of processed and out-of-season foods, we can have a varied and abundant diet that is available on a wide scale to most civilised countries today. However, with advancement of food technology and food processes, we can also have foods that are not entirely suitable for certain constitutions. Nor in the best interests of every one's body and genetic makeup. We also have information regarding some foods that is insufficient and possibly misleading. This is not always deliberate, just the process of research and understandings of adapted foods and current health challenges in today's society.

There is an increasing understanding in health areas of the contributions of certain foods toward inflammation in the body. This is a major cause of pain and issues leading to serious disease. At the very least, it can compromise many people, particularly those with arthritic, diabetic, obesity and cancer histories in their family lines.

It is worth considering the diet and work toward reducing those foods that produce inflammation, or at the very least, contribute toward it. It is easy to test for one's self. Removing certain foods or types of food for a period of two to three weeks to clear it out of the body and gut, then trying the same food for a day only to see the effects on one's health and energy.

I know myself that developing arthritis and muscle weakness cleared when I removed these foods from my diet. However, being an "O" blood group, and having tried to be Vegan or Vegetarian didn't work for me, and weakened me considerably, so I keep high quality and organic meat and fish still in my diet.

If you suffer a pain disorder, it is helpful to discover for yourself that inflammatory foods aggravate the condition. Processed, packaged and over prepared foods will certainly contribute to ill-health and inflammation, though some folks cannot digest all raw foods as their gut and digestive system may have been compromised or damaged by stress, inflammation, incorrect nutrition or certain medications. If there are digestive problems, assimilation of nutrition will be affected and reduced, and the stomach will find it hard to digest certain foods, especially cold food, as the digestive enzymes will be too challenged. Warm added ingredients can take the chill off too-cold a salad, stewed apples can replace raw, and adding some Papaya and Mint enzymes or a good balanced spectrum of digestive enzymes can help settle and optimise many meals.

Here are some foods that are linked to inflammation:

Fast food is often guilty of many harmful oils, sugar and artificial sweeteners, food additives, and a whole host of nasty ingredients.

Fried foods (French fries, onion rings, potato chips, nachos, hamburgers, etc.).

Food additives: colours, flavour enhancers, stabilizers, preservatives, etc. Some of the main ones include sulphites, benzoates, and colouring. Additives numbering 220-225 (Sulphur products). Additives 1440-1444 (Gluten products).

Dairy products (yogurt, ice cream, cottage cheese, butter, cheese, etc.). The reasons dairy products are inflammatory are many and today's dairy products are packed with hormones, antibiotics, and other harmful ingredients so avoid them as much as possible. One source of research indicates up to 60% of humans cannot digest milk.

Organic and Free Range eggs are still okay for some people.

Wheat products. Wheat itself is highly acid-forming and inflammatory in the body. Worse, most wheat available now is genetically-modified (GM). Many serious health conditions are starting to be linked to GM wheat consumption. Added to this there is also an increasing risk of toxicity in the grains due to the use of Roundup and other toxic herbicides and weed-killers due to the cumulative effect of these dangerous toxins in the human body.

Gluten-containing grains. Gluten is found in most grains and is highly inflammatory. Choose grains or seeds like buckwheat, quinoa, or millet for safer baking.

White sugar and sweets, including soft drinks and sweetened juices. Recent research is showing that sugar is one of the most addictive substances you can use. It's also highly inflammatory. At the very least, reduce your sugar consumption and choose fruit as your "go to" food when you're craving something sweet.

Alcohol. Alcohol is high in sugar and is a toxic burden to the liver. It is best eliminated or at the very least used in moderation. It can also affect the adrenals, causing a surge of adrenaline into the body, or an sudden imbalance of hormones.

Coca-Cola. This famous brew contains ingredients that strip rust off steel – not good for the digestive system, and though you may get a high, you will also get a damaged liver and digestive system.

Meat (not wild-caught fish). You don't have to go vegetarian here although an *organic* plant-based diet tends to be much lower in inflammatory substances but meat and poultry tend to cause some inflammation, so make them the background of meals, not the main dish.

Common Cooking Oils. Common vegetable cooking oils used in many homes and restaurants have very high omega-6 fatty acids and dismally low omega-3 fats. A diet consisting of an imbalanced omega-6 to omega-3 ration can promote inflammation and breed inflammatory diseases like heart disease and cancer.

Avoid Polyunsaturated vegetable oils such as grape seed, cottonseed, safflower, corn and sunflower oils. These industrial vegetable oils are also commonly used to prepare most processed foods and takeaways.

Replace your omega-6-saturated cooking oils with macadamia oil, extra virgin olive oil (not for cooking), or other edible oils with a more balanced omega-6 to omega-3 fatty acids ratio. Macadamia oil, for instance, has an almost one-to-one ratio of omega-6:3 fats, and it is also rich in oleic acid, a heart-healthy, monounsaturated fatty acid.

Canola Oil – This oil generally now comes from genetically modified sources and was developed from rapeseed to be more resistant to herbicide. Its ultimate usage and effects on the human body is still not guaranteed as safe. Only use if organic and definitely non-GMO guaranteed.

Anti-Inflammatory Foods:

Here is a list of foods that have anti-inflammatory properties. Not everyone can take everything, so experiment with what works for you.

Consider including in your diet as often as possible;

> Green Tea
>
> Pistachios
>
> Kiwi Fruit
>
> Tomatoes
>
> Olive Oil
>
> Green Leafy Vegetables, such as Spinach, Kale, and Collards
>
> Nuts like Almonds and Walnuts
>
> Fatty Fish like Salmon, Mackerel, Tuna, and Sardines
>
> Fruits such as Strawberries, Blueberries, Cherries, and Oranges
>
> Chia Seeds
>
> Turmeric
>
> Kim Chi
>
> Coconut Oil
>
> Cabbage
>
> Daikon Radish
>
> Kale

Mercury Toxicity

Mercury Toxicity can be acquired from a number of sources. These can include eating shellfish and larger varieties of fish. A highly toxic form (methylmercury) builds up in fish, shellfish and animals that eat fish. Mercury is also contained in some of the products we use, which may be found in consumer products in the home, burning coal, light bulbs, batteries, some paints, and used to be common in newsprint.

Dental amalgams are a major source of mercury toxicity. When you chew on them, they release minute emissions of toxic gases which are breathed in to the lungs and brain, as well as the digestive system. Over time, though dentists do not readily tell you, these amalgam fillings not only shrink, allowing further decay around the edges, but they also crack and deteriorate, and as they do so, your digestive system and intestinal lining takes the initial impact, until it travels through the body, ending up in the gut, the jaw, the brain or a myriad of other possible collection places. And the body does not get rid of it easy for it is cumulative in the body.

For many years dentists in Australia, England, and other major countries have continued to use dental amalgams for fillings in teeth, despite requests and warnings by natural health professionals.

Dental amalgams contain several toxic ingredients, the worst amongst them being **mercury**, which is highly toxic to humans, as well as being non-degradable and environmentally dangerous.

I first became aware of the danger of amalgams when I heard that Sweden was banning its use in their country in

1995. Mercury amalgam restorative material generally contains 50% mercury in a complex mixture of copper, tin, silver, and zinc. It has been well documented that the mixture in amalgams continually emits Hg (mercury - mercuric oxide) vapor, which is dramatically increased by chewing, eating, brushing, and drinking hot liquids. This is absorbed by the body via the tongue and absorbed into the digestive tract and system.

Health insurance stopped paying for amalgam restorations in Sweden in 1999. Since then, they have banned all mercury products making it illegal. Denmark and Norway now have a similar ban making it illegal since 2008-9. The American Dental Association has persistently said for the past 150 years that the mercury in amalgam is safe and does not leak. However, no clinical studies were ever done and the Food and Drug Administration approved amalgam under a grandfather clause. Subsequent studies have shown this claim of safety not to be true. Six states in the United States have enacted legislation that requires that informed consent brochures be given to the patient in a dental office before dental restoration in undertaken.

It is strongly linked to Multiple Sclerosis and has been demonstrated to have damaging effects on the kidney, central nervous system (CNS), and cardiovascular system, and has also been implicated in gingival tattoos. (In one study, the scientists concluded that amalgam Hg levels in kidney were sufficient to significantly decrease the rate of insulin clearance by non-defined mechanisms, and that electrolyte patterns in the urine were consistent with impaired renal tubular re-absorption.)

In another comprehensive experimental study by Lorscheider et al. they examined the effects of Hg (mercury) exposure upon cell function in the brain and in the intestinal bacteria. In rats, they demonstrated that ADP-ribosylation of tubulin and actin brain proteins was markedly inhibited, and that ionic Hg can thus alter a neurochemical reaction involved with maintaining neuron membrane structure. In monkeys, they showed that Hg, specifically from amalgam, will enrich the intestinal flora with Hg-resistant bacterial species which in turn also become resistant to antibiotics.

In short, it is a dread poison that the body usually cannot overcome, and it accumulates in the tissues, often in the kidneys, gastrointestinal tract and the jaw. Though it can gather in any part of the human body, some being known to gather in the brain and even joints.

Personal Mercury Toxicity Recovery

I personally had a health crisis through the use of these dangerous amalgams, and it took me a while to recover yet I am free from mercury toxicity now.

How did I do it?

Initially I did a clearing – using the techniques of kinesiology and working on the physical level as well as energetically with a therapist, we worked on supporting my kidney function to enable safe support during the mercury detoxification process. I also increased my Vitamin C intake to 4,000mcg (4 gms day) as a medicinal dose, increased my pure water consumption, and tried Hydrolated (or Hydrated) Bentonite. The Bentonite was effective to some degree, but I found that putting myself on a certain type of Chlorella was the key to it for me. This better purified and alkalized my blood and also fed the kidneys and other organs (liver especially) with nutritional supplements and herbs which also helped to support the process as the Chlorella flushed the mercury out - it seemed to bind itself to the stuff and so move it out of the body.

This meant starting off at a dose of 4 (tiny) little Chlorella tablets twice a day with a large glass of water, and increasing it by one extra tablet a day until I was taking ten tablets twice a day.

This strengthened and prepared my body to be better able to handle any toxic stir-up and release through attempting to remove the fillings.

I did this for a week then over a period of time I gradually had my amalgams replaced one by one, the worst leaking one removed first. Giving several months time between each session of amalgam replacement with a composite filling allowed the body to clear out what was stirred up with the drilling into the old mercury filling. I also used a dentist who employed an oxygen gas mask for me during fillings as well as a protective rubber gum "dam" which was fitted around the tooth to isolate and to collect any amalgam debris in order to prevent the tongue absorbing the bits of filling as it was being dug out.

My dentist at the time was amazing, and she had a special machine that measured the degree of mercury and toxic leakage from each tooth, in order to give the best program for removal. We could remove the worst first, and over time, improve my health overall and sufficiently to remove the next most toxic tooth amalgam for replacement with a compatible composite filling. Unfortunately, she was called away interstate due to family issues before the program was completed.

So I sought out another dental practitioner. One dentist had been highly recommended to me, and so I want along for a check-up and to see if he was suitable for completing my amalgam removal program. At the initial checkup, and after describing the need for a rubber dam and the precautions required for safe amalgam removal, he had seemed to already know about the procedure and to fully understand what was required as he agreed with me to all of this. I also explained that I would be recommending others to him for similar treatment.

When it came time for my next removal and replacement and I visited him for my next filling, I was thinking that he had fully understood the requirements as we had spent some time talking about it. I was astounded to find that before I had realized it, he did not do any of this, and had already completed digging out the old amalgam before I had realized what he had done. I felt little bits of old amalgam on my tongue, but thought that as I was clearing myself out I would be ok. But during the drilling, the friction of the drill released mercuric gases and I had no way of avoiding inhaling this in. Believing in the power of positive thought and strength of mind, I resolved that I would not let this affect me, and as I was still on the Chlorella it would all be managed. Though I was very disappointed with what he had done, and told him that I was surprised he hadn't used the dam and mask as discussed.

The reality of what had actually happened came later, as at the time, I thought, well he made a mistake, but I have reminded him and it should be ok next time.

Not so.

I got to see how dangerous this stuff really was for real - I was sick for six weeks after this – stomach cramps, feeling like crap, no energy, miserable. I bluntly refused to go back to him or recommend him again. And I told him why.

Eventually the Vitamin C and Chlorella (Sun-Chorella I found was the best for me to work with) cleared my system out and my energy began to return to me again.

Meanwhile, I had to repair and rebuild.

Hydration function is so important with this sort of toxicity clearing. The therapy that worked best for me and for others who I have helped with this problem were Hydration formats used in some branches of kinesiology. A good kinesiologist, or TCM practitioner will be able to help the kidneys to function better until the toxic Hg crap is cleared from the cells and body.

You will be surprised at how well you will feel after safe and ordered removal of amalgams and clearing their accompanying toxicity! Especially if you have been suffering Chronic Fatigue, MS or Leaky Gut (or Irritable Bowel Syndrome).

Oh, one word. I found a dentist who could measure which fillings are the worst or leaking the most (amalgams leak toxically with hot liquids and food as well as crack or shrink over time). This type of holistic dentist can measure the mercury leakage and tell you which fillings are the worst offenders to remove first. Don't forget to do it over a period of time, as each removal or change of filling can stir up the toxicity in the blood and body again and requires some clearing out or you may well overload with a toxic crisis.

Vitamins and minerals also play a very important part in toxicity removal and normal healthy functioning.

Vaccinations

Of late, there has been much controversy of the toxins used in vaccinations.

The Measles vaccine debate is still going strong, and was preceded with the eBola scare which seemed to blow over quite quickly. The Measles vaccine is included with a number of other vaccines for simultaneous inoculation. Given that Measles was once a simple illness consisting of just a few days at home, and which resulted in life-long immunisation, families in the 'old days' actually practised Measles Parties so that they could introduce Measles in a controlled and safe way to gain this advantage. It was once seen as a simple illness and necessary for immunity preparation. Leastways this was so when I was growing up.

The fact that extremely rare though it was as a cause of death, there is currently a huge outcry and demand for every parent to have their child inoculated. This is not surprising as since the introduction of the vaccine, Measles cases have actually increased and spread, and over time is becoming more virulent and resistant. These is a mistaken understanding that the Measles outbreaks were caused by non-vaccinated children, whereas in actual fact, those that have been vaccinated are actually suffering from the disease, often in a more destructive form and are in fact infecting others whether vaccinated or not.

False information on vaccines seems to reign and there is even evidence that there are programs for population reduction inherent in some of the vaccines being provided 'free'. This is a highly charged topic and debate, and there is insufficient space and time to enter into it here. However, I put forward these aspects for you to consider in the case of yours or a family member's health, particularly in the case of children. Vaccines are laden with 'carriers', preservatives, adjutants and a variety of other poisons and toxins. In some quarters there is overwhelming proof of connection with a compromised health, whilst in others there are strong denials. Uncovering links, agendas and business interests behind these is difficult, so you must make up your own mind. However, be aware that your local doctor may not have all the facts, and if you to investigate or do your own research, it is best to keep an open mind to arrive at your own truth.

It was little known that generally GP's or general practitioners of medicine were provided with minimum information regarding the ingredients of inoculations and vaccinations. The medical profession itself appears highly ignorant of what happens in the vaccination process, generally accepting and perpetuating the reasons provided when given their short introductory course instructions on how to administer them. Very few doctors have actually taken time out to read and study the provided documentation with the batches of vaccine, and very few have considered any of the ingredients. Busy as they can claim to be, and may in fact be, when *thinking*-doctors discover that among the components in vaccines there are some of the items I list shortly, they have been reported to not only be surprised and amazed, but also very concerned. In fact, some anti-vax doctors have totally 'disappeared' in America…

I have done some of my own research on this and believe the following to be an accurate picture of current pharma and vaccine activities. Some sites are listed at the end of the book. Here is a direct quote on the need for more care regarding vaccines.

"As the vaccine debate continues to go on, more and more people realize that yes, we do have to question the current state of our vaccines. I proposed a week ago that instead of looking at the vaccine argument as pro or anti vaccine, for now, let us look at it as something we need to keep exploring with an open mind so that we can make vaccines safer and better for those who choose to use them. I believe we all should have a choice in what we put in our bodies and many people are choosing not to vaccinate, not because they are crazy but because they truly have concerns. Unfortunately these concerns are not being addressed as well as they should be. Just as we don't want to turn a blind eye to potential disease, we can't turn a blind eye to the injuries happening because of vaccines.

That being said, when the government creates laws that protect vaccine manufacturers from being sued by families who have been injured by vaccines, and when you realize that $2,550,640,666.73 ($2.5 billion) has been paid out in compensation over the last 23 years due to vaccine injuries, you start to realize that yes, one size does not fit all when it comes to vaccines and they do have associated dangers. We should be re-visiting vaccine ingredients, schedules and necessity before we continue vaccinating the way we do. Do the benefits outweigh the risks?" (From http://www.collective-evolution.com/2014/01/28/you-want-to-vaccinate-my-child-no-problem-just-sign-this-form/ 2015)

This is a list of most of the ingredients found in children's vaccinations and vaccines in general, often comprised of the following chemicals, excipients, preservatives and fillers:

aluminum hydroxide

aluminum phosphate

ammonium sulphate

amphotericin B

animal tissues: pig blood, horse blood, rabbit brain,

arginine hydrochloride

dog kidney, monkey kidney,

dibasic potassium phosphate

chick embryo, chicken egg, duck egg

calf (bovine) serum

betapropiolactone

fetal bovine serum

formaldehyde

formalin

gelatine

gentamicin sulphate

glycerol

human diploid cells (originating from human aborted fetal tissue)

hydrocortisone

hydrolized gelatine

mercury   thimerosol   (thimerosal, Merthiolate(r))

monosodium glutamate (MSG)

monobasic potassium phosphate

neomycin

neomycin sulphate

nonylphenol ethoxylate

octylphenol ethoxylate

octoxynol 10

phenol red indicator

phenoxyethanol (antifreeze)

potassium chloride

potassium diphosphate

potassium monophosphate

polymyxin B

polysorbate 20

polysorbate 80

porcine (pig) pancreatic hydrolysate of casein

residual MRC5 proteins

sodium deoxycholate

sorbitol

thimerosal

tri(n)butylphosphate,

> VERO cells, a continuous line of monkey kidney cells, and washed sheep red blood

The really toxic and dangerous substances that I am aware of are in bold. There may be others in the list, and this is where your own research can help you to make informed decisions.

Now given that tests have been done for a period of three months on mice understood to aim at the reactions of the general population, there has been no released research on developing children UNDER twelve, nor on infants who have absolutely NO protection with the blood-brain barrier for the protective coating of the brain has not yet formed. Insufficient research is generally provided and the thinking has been that a three months research program is sufficient.

However, it is thought that many pharma companies request a 'fast-track' to a vaccine when they claim that it is necessary or essential for a current 'threatened' outbreak or possible danger of outbreak after they have the three months mandatory research. When the vaccine is approved, though, all further research is dropped and long-term effects, or other possible negative research or consequences are ignored, shelved, dropped or avoided.

Another currently hot issue on mercury toxicity is that even though it is a declared poison and doctors themselves declare that it should not be touched in any form, this deadly poison is actually in the very vaccinations given not just to adults, who have a better chance of fighting off their disastrous impact on the brain and the immune system, but to babies that are only weeks old. The climb in autism since pre-vaccination times is phenomenal, and is set to increase. Autism is just one of the new collateral on the pharmaco pushes of dictates in major so-called civilized countries. Given the amount of toxic chemicals in any given vaccine, and the fact that not one doctor is prepared to issue a guarantee of "no-harm" with any vaccine, one has to wonder what is really behind this current demand for all to conform. With much research demonstrating that non vaccinated children are faring better than vaccinated, and the growing research proving that vaccines actually do not give the protection that they promise, it is only a matter of time before an educated population exercises their choices and their *right* to their choices.

What to do about it

If you feel or find that there has been a history of many vaccines, and any reactions to them then I would think it wisest to focus on repairing the immune system. This can be through TCM, Herbs, acupuncture etc. Damaged nerves could possibly be assisted in the same way, but I would also investigate whether chiropractic, kinesiological, and the neuro sciences can aid in re-aligning or educating the neural systems themselves.

One thing I think is definitely worth looking at, and that is dietary support, including the Sun Chlorella tablets which can help in drawing out the toxic heavy metals from the blood and eventually the brain.

Re-establishment of correct hydration and also correct digestive and cellular assimilation can be supported with the right kinesiologist or therapist.

Minerals and Vitamins

It is surprising the number of people who understand the need for vitamins in their food. But there is often some vagueness when it comes to minerals.

I personally had to learn that all the vitamins that I was taking were simply expensive fluff going through my body as the body requires minerals to process the vitamins!

Vitamins need Minerals

Yes! I was surprised... But it's true. Minerals are required to process vitamins!

Minerals are required for proper body function, as the body cannot do its tasks without a sufficient uptake of the correct minerals. We are each comprised of minute quantities of minerals, and water requires these for so many processes in the body.

There are many minerals that we require, but I will take a quick look at those that are the most common and therefore the quickest to get depleted and overlooked.

Most minerals come from plants and must be grown in a mineral-rich soil in order to contain the essential minerals need by the human body. Some minerals come indirectly from animal sources. Other minerals may come from certain types of water.

List of Important Minerals:

The major minerals are potassium, magnesium, calcium, sulfur, phosphorus, sodium and chloride. The trace minerals are zinc, iron, iodine, selenium, copper, manganese, fluoride, chromium, manganese and molybdenum. Trace minerals are also important for human growth and development but they are required in smaller amounts than the major minerals.

Calcium requires other minerals for correct utilization or it can build up and form calcifications on bones.

Magnesium is involved in 300 essential metabolic reactions in the human body, such as energy production, synthesis of essential molecules, structural roles, ion transport across cell membranes, cell signaling and cell migration. Magnesium deficiencies are on the rise due to general farming practices and over-processing of important magnesium-rich foods such as beans, nuts, whole grains and green leafy vegetables.

Potassium supports fluid balance in the body and is the principal positively charged ion or cation in cell fluid, with sodium being the cation outside the cells. The delicate balance of this interaction of sodium and potassium is important to 'sustaining life' and is critical for nerve impulse transmission, muscle contraction and heart function.

The trace minerals **iron** and **zinc** are also extremely important minerals for the health of the human being. Iron metabolizes other nutrients, regulates growth and supports the immune system. Iron helps in 'the formation of red blood cells and facilitates oxygen transportation throughout the body'.

Zinc is an antioxidant involved in normal immune function, wound healing and sexual development, with a supporting role for the liver. It is critical for the body's defence against allergies and viruses. Severe zinc deficiency affects the stomach PH balance, affecting assimilation of all minerals even including zinc itself. An energy balance can help to correct this.

Phosphorus is important for healthy bones and teeth, it is found in every cell and is part of the system that maintains acid-base balance.

The best source of **sodium** that I have found is through Himalayan or Pink Salt, which is rich in natural minerals. I also use a mineral rich solution that I add to water and is pleasant citrus tasting drink. This is called Citramin and is filled with Full-spectrum plant and sea derived colloidal minerals.

This means that it is easily absorbed by the body without any gut irritation. I was using another colloidal mineral solution, but there were still tiny bits and particles that floated in the suspension, which did cause me some irritation. I stopped using it because it had not been dissolved enough and aggravated my already sensitive digestion. Citramin is the only mineral solution not in a see-through bottle that I will use – I won't use any other colloidal mineral brand unless it is in a clear bottle so that I can see if there are any bits floating in it. Experiment and find your own minerals as there are plenty of balanced solutions out there. But please do include it in your diet, even if you only add it every other day.

Magnesium:

Magnesium is the number one mineral that tends to get overlooked and yet this is required in the largest amount by the body. Especially for hydration.

It is effective for muscle twitches and cramps as well as being so important for nerve transmission, immune system health and making protein in the body. Increase in magnesium can have an almost immediate effect.

On top of my multi-mineral mix, I add further magnesium because through being a Sensitive I had found that I need more of it than non-sensitive people. It is best to supplement with a magnesium chelate or oratate, or similar.

Magnesium Phosphate Schuessler Salts has assisted some cases of arthritis pain within minutes when placed under the tongue to assimilate via the bloodstream, but this has usually been after the kidneys energy flow has been corrected – in kinesiology sessions.

Magnesium chloride is not easily assimilated and therefore wasteful to take internally, though it is very effective when added to bath water or applied topically to aching parts of the body.

It can be made up or bought as Magnesium Oil (or Nigari) and its absorption is a lot faster than waiting for a supplement to take effect. Sensitive skins may require a cream beforehand, or instead use one made up as Schuessler Tissue Salts Cream – Mag Phos (Magnesium Phosphate).

A word here – it is best assimilated before 6pm.

Magnesium Deficiency Causes

Magnesium deficiency can be caused by the following:

- Sugar Excess – robs the body of magnesium
- Mercury amalgam dental fillings
- Excess dairy foods
- Too much caffeine – coffee, tea, chocolate
- Not enough leafy green vegetables or fruit
- Non-organic food
- Too much processed food
- Smoking
- Alcohol excess
- Stress
- Jaw muscle (temporalis) under tension
- Unresolved Trauma
- Excess calcium
- Intense exercise

An even bigger problem than magnesium deficiency is the inability to utilize magnesium. This is usually caused by kidney tension, and is often present in major health problems.

Magnesium Symptoms

Magnesium deficiency triggers or causes the following conditions; the introduction of magnesium, either by a high-magnesium diet, with green drinks, or magnesium supplements, can help alleviate these conditions:

- Anxiety and panic attacks
- Asthma
- Backaches
- Blood clots
- Body-tension

- Bowel disease
- Bruxism (jaw clenching)
- Chronic Fatigue
- Constipation
- Chocolate, caffeine cravings
- Cystitis
- Depression
- Detoxification
- Diabetes, Syndrome X, & Metabolic Syndrome
- Fatigue
- Heart disease, disorders
- Hypertension
- Hypoglycemia
- Insomnia
- Kidney Disease
- Liver Disease
- Migraine
- Musculoskeletal conditions
- Nerve problems
- Osteoporosis
- Raynaud's Syndrome
- Tooth decay

An amazing list of issues, and all linked to magnesium... How come the role of this valuable, indeed essential mineral, has not been fully recognized by the medical profession?

It may well be because only one percent of magnesium in the body is distributed in the blood, thus making a simple sample of magnesium in a blood test highly inaccurate and therefore almost irrelevant as a reliable test.

This is probably why most doctors who rely on blood tests for magnesium and who don't check for or are not aware of the magnesium deficiency signs and symptoms, and who also probably do not realise that up to 80 percent of the population is deficient, will miss an important diagnosis.

If you have a serious health problem I can recommend "The Miracle of Magnesium" by Carolyn Dean.

Magnesium Rich Foods

Below is a list of high magnesium foods, in order of nutrient density:

- Dark Leafy Greens; Raw Spinach, Swiss Chard, Kale
- Nuts and Seeds; Squash and Pumpkin Seeds, Sesame Seeds, Brazil Nuts, Almonds, Cashews, Pine Nuts, Mixed Nuts, Peanuts, Pecans
- Fish; Mackerel, Pollock, Turbot, Tuna, Most Other Fish
- Whole Grains; Brown Rice, Quinoa, Millet, Bulgur, Buckwheat, Wild Rice, Whole Wheat, Barley, Oats
- Beans And Lentils; Soy Beans, White Beans, French Beans, Black-Eyed Peas, Kidney Beans, Chickpeas, Lentils, Pinto Beans
- Avocados
- Low-Fat Dairy; Plain Non Fat Yogurt, Goat Cheese, Nonfat Chocolate Yogurt
- Bananas
- Dried Figs
- Dark Chocolate

Zinc

As one of the most important essential minerals, zinc is involved in hundreds of vital enzymatic reaction in the body. It is called an essential trace element because small amounts are necessary for overall health. Zinc is basically a mineral/metal and has a high affinity for electrons – this enables interactions with several amino acid side chains. Some of the critical roles it appears to be involved in are:

- Regulating gene expression and supporting healthy cellular growth
- Maintaining a normal sense of taste and smell
- Promoting healthy eyes
- Supporting immune function and maintaining a healthy metabolic rate

Zinc is an essential trace mineral with more biological roles than all other trace elements combined, yet the body cannot manufacture it nor can it store it.

Some of the food sources containing zinc include:

- Liver
- Crimini mushrooms
- Spinach and sea vegetables
- Oysters
- Pumpkin seeds
- Beef
- Green peas
- Raw milk and cheese
- Beans

And if you are eating these yet not getting the benefit, it is because it is over-processed or over-cooked.

An oral taste test can quickly tell you if you are deficient, by using the Zinc Tally Test at home or in your healthcare specialists clinic or office. Zinc Tally can be purchased at certain health stores or from health practitioners. Other tests include;

- Serum test – not entirely accurate
- Plasma test – may be insensitive to marginal deficiencies
- Tolerance test – measures changes after taking zinc orally
- Hair test – generally most often used by natural medicine doctors

Zinc is vital to your health to:

- Maintain healthy bold sugar levels
- Regulate protein synthesis
- Support a healthy respiratory system
- Promote healthy cell functioning and division (growth and repair)
- Support a normal-functioning GI tract
- Protect against oxidative distress
- Support ageing

Vegetarians in particular should ensure that they are taking sufficient zinc in their diet. And it is always best to get advice from a health professional regarding the type of zinc supplement and the quantity as zinc comes in several forms – Zinc Gluconate, Zinc Amino Acid Chelate, and Zinc Citrate. And sometimes (more often than not) all forms are required.

Zinc deficiency or low zinc supplies can exacerbate the effects of stress on the body as well. It has also been linked to hair loss as well as skin and nails. And low libido.

Because it affects the sense of smell and taste, low zinc can also lead to cravings for saltier or sweeter foods.

Zinc Deficiency Symptoms

- Low energy
- Chronic fatigue
- Infertility
- Poor immunity
- Bad memory
- Inability to focus
- Slow wound healing
- Nerve dysfunction
- Ringing in the ears
- Apparent ADD symptoms
- Diarrhea

So when looking at low energy and compromised nutrition, check your diet for sufficient zinc and your body for correct assimilation.

Before Self Medication or Self Treatment

Always seek the advice or guidance of a professional or expert. Again look to a TCM practitioner, Naturopath, Homeopath, Kinesiologist who has studied anatomy or hydration (amazing results this way).

Having said that, there is nothing wrong with putting yourself on a healthy regime, opting for fresh or organic foods, reducing the amount of toxic fats – not all fats, they are essential for healthy function – increasing your fresh fruit and vegetables, reducing processed foods, additives and preservatives, and in finding many other balanced ways of improving your nutritional intake.

But some people may approach this too radically and think that they can speed things up by resorting to a new herb they have heard of – for they may well not realize the power that there is in herbal remedies.

Please do only take herbs such as gingko biloba, gotu kola or other strong herbs advisedly and carefully, as you must deal with the body as a whole, and sometimes too much stimulation in the wrong organ, gland or system at the wrong time can damage rather than aid the healing process.

I have known many to self medicate. If you stimulate, say, the liver, to do a detox program, and the lymphatic system is in distress, you will overload the lymphatic system and have a health crisis. There is no point in putting yourself in bed for weeks unnecessarily in the attempt to get healthier...

Sensitives always need to be more careful as their systems can respond or react very quickly to too much of something, so always begin with a reduced doseage of anything and gradually increase it.

If you are ultrasensitive and have a compromised adrenal system, then an unsupervised liver cleansing may well be too much for your energy systems to cope with.

Even too strong a massage can put an extra strain on the body. A bit like that familiar hotel story again, though this time it's like clearing out and redecorating several major rooms at the same time yet still expecting everything to carry on as exactly as usual – not really possible.

Better to identify the correct or most appropriate detoxification pathways first, and to work out appropriately the order of healing or support that your body needs in order to regain proper function again, rather than to exacerbate the problem.

Excess Weight – a Word

When looking at losing excess fat, we may think that we just need to diet.

There are literally thousands of diets out in the world. A truth about weight-loss diets is that calories intake less calories exercised equals excess calories stored.

However, there *are* other circumstances that affect this simplified equation!

There are many reasons why the body retains weight, often depending on age, gender, life style, circumstances and history. If the weight is stubborn, and not just an apparent imbalance of too much food versus not enough exercise, then I suggest that you get a thorough check-out first with your local medic, complementary therapies doctor, Chinese medicine practitioner as well as energetic advise from your kinesiologist or bionutritionist. There could be hormonal issues, psychological or energetic issues or a combination of these that need to be addressed.

> **+ C IN – C OUT = C STORED x 'X'**
> **Calories In Less Calories Out Equals Calories Stored**
> **'X' Times Physical + Emotional Function**

We often assume it is the sorts of foods we eat that affects weight, and to quite a degree this is true. Assuming, of course, that our nutrition is being fully absorbed. It is always a good idea to check out the body's ability to digest and absorb properly. It may be creating cravings through faulty digestion and the inability to draw the energy from a 'normal' diet or its current diet. Mercury toxicity will have an impact on the intestines ability to absorb nutrition, and your body will be accumulating toxicity because it cannot use the nutrition it is being fed, and it is slow at removal of these unbroken down items – well usually it's because it doesn't have the energy to do so.

Imagine that hotel again – deliveries coming in daily, but the staff cannot open up or break-down the parcels of nutrition so they end up being side-lined whilst they try to open the next lot on the conveyor belt of life – in short a lot of parcels unopened begin cluttering up the passageways, and people are being slowed down in trying to get past them to go about their business. Everyone crying out for help because they can't do as much as they used to but they are expending more energy. And good old sugar, in any form, will often be forced to come to the rescue in order to get out of this 'sticky (pardon the pun) situation.

Sometimes then the weight is simply unprocessed nutrition that the body is having difficulty not only recognizing and using, but also disposing of the same.

I have seen people who cannot process gluten (which is particularly challenging to digest and absorb in its present GMO state) accumulate a lot of puffiness round their ankles. Sometimes the puffiness is lack of proper hydration – the kidney and liver meridians are along the ankles – and each function or lack of function can impact on the other.

Weight can also be caused by faulty processing of; thyroid, kidneys, liver, lymphatics, salivary glands, small and large intestine, bladder, gall bladder, adrenals, circulation, hormones and glandular system.

A new and emerging picture of **Leptin**-Resistance also provides another piece of the puzzle and a good nutritionist can lead you in the right direction for the best tests to ascertain this. Leptin is a major factor in satiety and metabolism.

Stress can play a huge part in weight issues, as can Thyroid related problems. When a trauma has been experienced, or a long term stress, it can compromise the adrenals whose job it is to produce hormones that get us going and keep us going. When they are continually aroused by dramas, crises and stress, they forget how to turn off – a bit like having a foot jammed on the accelerator in a car. And they also become exhausted. So that when you also have a foot on the brake – because you cannot change the situation or event and no longer have the energy to move forward from it – then you simply don't go anywhere, and you feel tired using all that fuel / juice up without taking action.

The fall-out from all of this, even when the stress is over or the trauma is buried, is that the body can still hold the excess cortisol from the adrenaline that flooded through and this can stay locked into the fat cells or other cells in the body. This can be very stubborn to move, and when one attempts to lose weight and release the toxins from the fat cells, the associated memories of stress may also be stirred up for release, which can emerge in a way that one feels the old emotions and stress all over again. Without knowing why.

This can sabotage attempts to continue the process. Or make one feel incapable of creating the change that they desire. The answer is to uncover the attached or hidden memory and deal with it in a way that prevents it affecting one again. Affirmations and energy work can really help with this.

So it is not necessarily wise to always assume that any calorie or carbohydrate-reduced diet will automatically fix weight increase or obesity. Not every fat person is fat simply because they are eating too much.

Besides the stress hormonal imbalances, there are also some further contributors such as these Psychological related issues that can be connected with weight issues.

Some of these could include –

- Self protection
- Fear of sexual abuse
- Fear of being noticed
- Taking on or absorbing others responsibilities or problems
- Lack of joy in life
- Stuffing down emotions especially anger
- And even just plain boredom.

Energetically, with the above issues, you may well find that the central and governing meridians will not be 'on' (that is they will not be functioning correctly) or nourished, and that the person often doesn't feel supported, or able to be who they truly are.

Spiritual disconnection or a sense of being lost or alone can also be the cause or the consequence of the above. A kinesiologist can check and help to correct this with you.

The back and nervous system are closely connected and one will and can affect the other. With weight issues, the back may well need attention, and there may be pain or stiffness at the hips or lower down the spine, at sometimes at the rear of the heart or at the neck and jaw. Sometimes all of these areas are affected.

The back represents feeling supported.

Finding a good chiropractor, osteopath, or someone who does Bowen Therapy or Cranio-Sacral work can also help. As well as dealing with the underlying emotional issues. Feeling that Life is not supporting us will often create back problems. Dealing with these fears or issues will allow the back a better chance to maintain itself.

Another factor and one that is often missed is this: How comfortable are we living in our body?

To extrapolate on this, let's go one step further...

How comfortable are we being in a human body, living on Planet Earth?

Some people are not at all comfortable, whilst others revel in it. Those that are not comfortable may find dealing with other people fraught with difficulties or misunderstandings. Getting more comfortable through self development, or for some, Soul healing, can assist them in this area.

So when asking yourself just "how comfortable..." you are and noting your own personal response may provide a further key, as to whether or not you belong to a group of more sensitive souls that can experience difficulty with how life is conducted in our current human society. For as mentioned, some often feel like they don't really want to be here on some level of their being, and as I have often heard from some, they simply "Want to go Home" – wherever Home may be...!

I have had this thought myself, so I know it can be a real issue for some. Learning to get comfortable about the reason one may possibly have chosen to be here, or learning to accept that we are indeed here (though usually this is after having to realize that possible resistance to being here has been behind some issues) can allow one to make better sense of life or of the events of life that we have experienced.

Focusing on our own inner integrity rather than the integrity (or lack of it) from others can help us to move forward and begin to create a better life experience. So this is really about our inner spirit, our spirituality, that inner flame or knowing deep inside.

And about hearing it and making it more comfortable...

PSYCHOLOGICAL BLOCKS TO HEALTH AND HEALING

We are amazing beings – our bodies are designed to always seek to fix problems and to function for us.

Sometimes however, it lacks the necessary raw repair materials, so will use whatever is available to it. It is amazing what a mechanic can do to get his car on the road again when out in the wild without the proper tools or brand new parts... or what the enterprising person when challenged can make do with using recycled materials.

The body and mind is able to shunt off energy for more needy areas, and to 'bury' toxic issues in order to deal with the job in hand – using its 'compensation' abilities and 'suppressing' the problems till better times allow it to deal with the problem. Or to use the analogy of the hotel again, it is amazing how one can shortchange the staff or the workers to provide for the requirements of the priority guests or essential tasks.

This can happen on both the physical level, and on the psychological level.

What often happens, though, is that the day of clearing or sorting out old buried stuff can be postponed, or indeed may not even arise, as we often simply take for granted that things are okay – 'the body / personality / mind is still functioning ok, so why bother?'

In essence we have learned to cope.

This is not the same as well-being or health. The lack of energy is because energy is tied up in maintaining this 'management', this 'compensation' or 'suppression'.

And this state will continue until we either collapse, reach a crisis point, or the issue erupts in our face, whether in a meltdown, depression or disease.

The Power of Thoughts and Words

Many people do not yet fully realise the power that is in the spoken word. Nor the power of our thoughts to create. Most of us have some understanding that when we intend to do something and we are single minded about it, then we have every chance to actually achieve the goal we have set, for we are determined to achieve it – if at all possible. No house or building is built without first conceiving it in the mind. Thoughts have power, and you can sometimes hear the predominant thoughts of many by what they say – positive people who think positively say positive things, and generally negative people who tend to think negatively generally say negative things.

How the predominance of thoughts arrived at being generally negative or generally positive is another story, and for me personally it was quite a journey to unravel from my own subconscious mind and heart the various negative things that had held me back. But I first had to arrive at the understanding that something needed to be changed within me.

Many years ago, after I had experienced a particularly devastating event, I came across a book by Florence Scovell-Schinn. It was called "Your Word is Your Wand". I was a serious Christian at the time, so was a bit uncertain about the "Wand" part, having been indoctrinated with anti-magic dogma. But Florence wasn't meaning it literally as a wand, but rather as a reference to recognising that your word had power to it. This was new to me, though I was aware of the biblical creation references to "The Word" which was certainly a mystical manifestation of word-power. Yet I continued on with her little book and it changed my life. Literally. I later joined a church group that recognized metaphors in the bible and this underscored what I was learning from this book.

The gist of her writings and philosophy was that our word actually has a power. When we speak with truth and focus, we can create. This may sound a bit strange to some people, but when someone you know personally and that never lies says something, you know that you can count on their "word" being their word and that what they say they mean. This also means that you respect their word and this brings them a certain kind of power. And when they truly intend something and commit to it, then it will be done!

Not so with lots of people that we all know who say things that suit them at the time, whose words can be wishy-washy, and who never really achieve what they say they will, not matter how convincing they try to sound. They are generally wishy-washy people. Their words lack power and conviction, because they have watered them down with half-intentions, with a proliferation of insincere words and followed these words up with non-action.

I call them "the shoulda, woulda, coulda's" – I should have done this..., I could have done that..., I would have done the other... etc, but they never do and probably are not capable to do. And when they genuinely want something to happen, the things they talk about don't come to pass because they talk all the energy and soul out of it mainly through bragging or attempts at impressing which loses the power of their word in extraneous posturing – it becomes "all talk". Whereas it is a different story for the ones who watch their words, for they are often the ones who say little and who merely hint at something yet it comes to pass.

So the power of our word can become quite strong when we are mindful of following them up with action and intent consistently.

But there is also another part to the equation and that is also the content of our word once it is strong and meaningful.

For the predominance of our words, just like our thoughts, influences our life and experience of life as well as possibly limiting our life. A good friend of mine discovered that she had a brain tumour. I attempted to let her know what I knew about the power that words had to be fulfilled, but she didn't understand what I was trying to say. A woman with a big heart, it was not my place to "fix" her, just to support her choices. But I must confess every time when something went wrong for her that she had a struggle with she would declare: "It's doing my head in!" And so it was, quite literally. It did her head in; with a tumour.

Another friend was in the habit of saying how much she needed a break, and sure enough, the break came – she broke her leg seriously in two separate places. I saw this with two other friends, and even though I suggested that instead they declare "I would really like a rest" instead, it wasn't until they got their "break" that they twigged what they had been asking for. In fact, two of them said to me "I will be more careful of what I ask for now, for I obviously got it." As a matter of fact, this same thing had happened to me earlier for I had broken my writing and doing arm whilst complaining that I had needed a break – and so I learned this lesson the hard way – *"Be careful what you wish for, for you might get it!"*

If we have the power of creating something like this that can affect us so drastically, might it not be an interesting exercise to hear what we say to ourselves and others, and see what we have created with our words (and thoughts) and maybe be more mindful of better choices of what we wish for in our lives?

A truth in life is that when we become mindful of our words and our thoughts, we are in a better place to learn how to change them and of how to use them. This can often change our experience of life and improve our health.

When we want to get well, but we don't really think we can, then whatever it is that we really think, that can well become our truth and experience. There is a saying: *What you think you can do, you can.* If you don't believe you can, then you won't. One first has to conceive of something to create it.

Don't limit yourself, be determined to discover the answers to your issues and to embrace a better way, and you have already given yourself a head start (so to speak).

The section on Affirmations may give you more inspiration on creating or choosing different realities and experiences for your life.

Positive Energy

We live in a sea of energy. Science is discovering that all is made of energy, and all things vibrate to their own particular and unique frequencies. Working with the frequency of the spoken word, with the frequency projected out into the realm of the unseen by thought, you are projecting out a particular frequency, and this frequency can have the power to change the existing frequency to a better or healing frequency.

We have all felt the healing power of someone's genuine words of care or love, as we have negative frequencies clothed in words to hurt.

When we hold a frequency of illness, stress or dis-ease in the body, consider how to change the frequency with not only the right knowledge, nutrition and ability to process these nourishing things, but also with the right healing frequency. We have talked about the power of nature to heal; that is the power of the healing frequencies of nature to heal. Consider the healing frequencies of sound, of colour, of ambience, of positive words, of positive thoughts.

Your thoughts really matter - the way you think matters. You are a broadcasting tower of vibrational frequencies and by changing the way you think about things you can change your results. When you think a new thought, or entertain a new dream, or mentally choose a new goal, your thoughts "leave" you and go out – unseen and in every direction.

These ripples affect the current frequencies and can change your current situation.

So pay attention at what you are putting out into your life, and into your reality, as well as what is coming in from others.

Choose those frequencies and energies and words and thoughts that support you and your health and your well-being. This way, you will be able to take charge of your life and your health.

Reasons Not to Change and Heal

With so much external 'noise' and activity around us, it is often hard to hear the inner promptings or whispers of things not being 'quite right'.

There are also times when it suits us to ignore the promptings – Such as when:

- We don't want to change
- We get a spin off benefit for things being the way they are
- We want to blame someone or something else for our state
- We get to be taken care of
- We don't have to or want to take responsibility
- We get to complain and get attention
- Behind it all we feel the need to 'punish' ourself or someone else
- It supports our belief that the world 'sucks', 'doesn't care', 'life is crap' or whatever else we want to hold onto

To get well, we have to not only be truly willing to do so, we have to be willing to change, and to let go of what we have been holding on to. We have to release our inner conflict, between aspects or parts of ourself that want different outcomes.

The head may want to get better, but the heart may want to stay hurt. Or hold onto whatever else the hidden pain or issue is. All of this requires a shift in our attitude and a genuine examination of whether we truly want to get well - to dare to risk a change in our present situation.

Challenging your inner thoughts will give you clues as to what is going on.

You may have to listen carefully, for they often run through the mind so quickly like lightning, leaving only their impression behind; but try to do it anyway. You do get better at it with time.

Or work with a counselor, therapist, kinesiologist or other to uncover your own hidden truths.

Understanding yourself is one of the great gifts you can give yourself.

I do not know of anybody who lies in bed in the morning deciding that they will be the worst version of who they are that day. Most of us simply do the best we can.

The greatest gift though is to love yourself.

Then you can begin to accept and respect yourself, and move toward being the best you that you can be.

A Word on Spirituality

As we are more than just our body, more than just our emotions, more than just our mind, and indeed we are a combination of all of these things – most of us now recognize that we are also a spirit, an inner intelligence and observer. So it is fitting that we have a quick look at what this means and how this impacts on one's health.

The word 'Spirituality' is so often been confused with 'Religion', 'Faith', 'Church' / 'Synagogue' / 'Temple' and even 'Psychics' and 'Mediums'.

These are NOT necessarily about Spirituality!

Generally speaking religion is about tradition; faith is about what we want to believe; church etc. is about formal socializing or grouping connected with a religion; psychics are about extrasensory perceptions, and mediums are about accessing unseen beings and entities. Some of these labels and practices may be associated with spirituality. All of these may also be associated with Power. But does not define them necessarily as 'spiritual'. Yes, belief definitely comes into it – our choices of any of these above expressions (of so-called 'Spirituality') reflecting our beliefs.

Spiritualism is also not necessarily spiritual in the application here – it tends to be more concerned with the unseen and the spirits rather than the spirituality I am addressing here – that indefinable centre of each of us which can connect to the highest and the best, the purest and the divine.

I want to get really clear on this, because I have observed and experienced so much Spiritual Snobbery and hypocrisy that comes in the guise of 'holiness' and claimed in the name of 'God'. Usually, it has actually been hiding egotism, self-righteousness, arrogance, lack of compassion, downright prejudice, rudeness, the need to 'be right' or other major control issues.

Each and every one of us is a spiritual being – that is our inner essence. Whether a saint or sinner, priest or prostitute, thief or therapist, each of us has a unique and precious inner essence.

Of course, what we choose to do with this is another story. But let me continue.

> **Actions speak louder than words!**
> **'By their Fruits ye shall know them...'**

The person who attends his religious meeting house, and yet deliberately disadvantages, abuses or robs his fellow man, woman or a child is demonstrating his lack of real spiritual connection.

The person who gives to charity, yet takes advantage in his or her business dealings is showing his lack of internal spiritual completeness.

The person who avoids organized religion, who doesn't fit in with the beliefs of others, and yet has compassion and respect for his fellow man, is often much more in tune with his or her spirituality than those professing to be so.

I used to think that you were spiritual when you spoke, understood or used spiritual words, phrases, ideas and concepts. Time and maturity as well as life experience

114

has shown me that what we do and how we live often speaks more truly of who we really are. The challenge is to walk the talk!

When one's spirit has been cut off from what it feels or knows as the Highest Divine that there is, it can feel very lonely and isolated. When one is forced into a religion or cult or some system other than one that truly resonates with their spirit, it can be debilitating. I think that one of our life lessons is to find the truth of our own personal beliefs, our own personal conscience, and not something that we have been brought up with.

It's about being congruent, being in an inner integrity. Then there are no conflicting energies within our being, no inner conflict that will reveal itself in our body. Our inner spirit will have a harmony with our mind and emotions and this will naturally reveal itself in the body

.

What Is Spirituality Really?

I no longer count on the intellectual persuasion, language or arguments or charismatic bleatings of someone to impress or convince me that they are spiritual. I have met humble people that touch those around them with a truly healing heart. And I have met (and worked with) others professing themselves as 'Masters' and even 'Enlightened' working in all manner of positions and 'callings' who are egotistical, abusive, dangerous and manipulative, and some of who actually seem to suck the soul out of another to feed themselves. Some I have even called Twilight Masters because they have a little measure of Light but basically live and work with the Dark.

What I have discovered for myself is that the person who:

Acknowledges and appreciates nature and this planet

Treats him / her self and others with respect

Is mindful of how his / her actions affect others

Is who he says he is, with true integrity

Aspires to the highest in their life and expression, whilst accepting and whilst;

Seeking to understand their own nature

Acknowledges and honors the male energy and role, and

Protects and nurtures the female energy and role

Seeks to live in harmony

Has healthy boundaries and respects the boundaries of others

Aspires to be honest with him or herself and honest

Tends to act without harm to others

- is far more likely to be connected with their spirituality than anyone professing to have a 'fast-track' to God.

The psychic who thinks that they are spiritual simply because they have clairvoyance or some other gift needs to get clearer on just what spirituality really is, because it's not necessarily that!

Seeing angels doesn't make them one...

The person with any sort of 'Power' is deluding them self if they think that this puts them above others. Sure, they may have more knowledge (or 'more power'), but this does not make them 'better than', nor more entitled than!

Psychics and persons of religious authority or anyone with 'Power' are just people too. They can have problem relationships, difficult or 'bad-hair' days, and certainly do not have a monopoly on 'the truth'!

I have mixed with many psychics, and let me tell you that their spirituality does not rest upon their gifts or abilities.

Fortunately I have met some who are both psychic and spiritual, and who aspire to the highest outcomes possible. They have had to work on their ego, their pride, their integrity and their self honesty, for often their gifts got in the way.

But after doing so, they became real people and channels for great healing and change on the planet. And were a blessing to be with!

On Being 'Special'

So many people now seek to be 'Special'. This can be energetically wearing, as there is no doubt that each individual is already unique... for there is not another like them anywhere in the world. The problem with the struggle to be 'special' – often by seeking fame or celebrity of some sort – is that the personality needs to be admired or to gain the attention of others because it is so starved in itself, and in my opinion secretly feels inadequate.

The current trend of '15 minutes of fame', whether on TV, YouTube, internet postings or stupid acts to get newsworthy attention shows a real need for something that they are not giving, or not able to give, themselves. Sure I know that this can be used for marketing, to make money and sensation. It has a part in our world of social public access. And some things can be put on the internet quite innocently yet create a runaway sensation.

There is a huge difference between humility with accidental fame, and self-seeking notoriety. One has room for others, the other has only room for them self and sees the world as purely for their own disposal and service. Not a nice look.

For some of these self-seekers, a part of them desires that others 'see' them as something 'special' or different to avoid the personal effort of liking themselves or to avoid having to make peace on the inside.

In adolescence, with so much hormonal activity, and difficulty in putting on 'the brakes' when risk escalates to danger, as well as the inability of not seeing the consequences of actions fully, some attention seeking activities can even destroy lives.

And with the current media examples of how ordinary life appears to be, and the endless programs on murder, destruction and all things bad in life, it can be hard for the not-yet-adult to be able to recognise real life and reality. We live in a society of competition and of having to be the 'winner' rather than a 'loser' – which is not a healthy equation, for there can only be one winner. Instead of a cultivation of self competition where we look at how we can improve on ourself to be the best we can, we are encouraged to take a side and to win and also to want others to lose. This is the psychology of war not peace or unity, and is divisive. Our self image suffers if we 'lose' because the side we chose does not win.

It takes a lot of energy to try and be something that you are not. It takes far less energy to focus on being the best of who you can be. Placing others above your own inner voice and conscience is giving your power away.

It also contributes a portion of your energy towards that person, thereby allowing you less energy. Sometimes we need guidance to take us to our next level.

I have noted that the more 'normal' and 'ordinary' that a person with gifts aspires to be, the less of their ego gets in the way, and the more they are accessible to others. They become more 'Special' by virtue of their ordinariness or humanity.

The more that they try to be their true self, the more they shine. And the more others are drawn to them.

Remember not to let someone keep you back when you are ready to go on to another level, no matter who they are.

Sensitives

Sensitives (very sensitive or energetically aware types of people) are particularly prone to energy overwhelm, energy drains, or energy explosions, whether emotional, physical or mental. Like sponges, they tend to soak up not just atmosphere, but the toxins of others.

They need to take special care to nurture their inner core, as the stronger they become energetically, the easier to negotiate life.

They are like the early miner's canaries – they signal the first signs of problems.

Over-sensitivity is a very difficult life experience. Often, they struggle to be understood, and often don't understand themselves. What I have observed is that they usually have a special gift, but have not yet learned how to control or manage it.

Personally, I was quite sensitive as a child, and no one around me understood it. Over time I gradually saw that I was viewing it from a negative aspect, and hadn't seen the strength and the gift in it. I had thought it weakened me, but when I discovered that it actually gave me insight into people and their situations, and therefore benefited my work with others, then I was able to begin to work with it in a more expanded way.

My next necessary step was then to learn about my boundaries, and how to set them and monitor them. And this is tricky when they have been badly stepped upon. But doable.

Often Sensitives can be deeply wounded or are overly aligned to the pains of others.

When they can recognise that they are identified with this pain or whatever, and they are willing to release and give this up, and separate from the pain, they will begin to find the goodies and the hidden gifts. Though this may firstly require awareness of what their body consciousness is taking on, then learning how to work with that and overcome it by releasing it.

One of the challenges to succeed in this can be to discover (it is there, waiting) their own inner strength and power. Not power in the sense of overpowering others, as do bullies, control freaks or psychic manipulators (or as certain supposed 'psychic readers'). But the power to accept who they are, and that this is not necessarily negative, but a different kind of strength, and then stand up for oneself, rather than be overpowered or fear having to avoid any action that would put them at variance with another.

When they honor themselves this way, value their own contribution and find their own voice, they usually find they can more easily manage their sensitive-ness.

Positive Thought

We have often heard of the phrase 'Think Positive'. So many times I hear that the answer to life or problems in life is to think positively. Easy to do when everything is going well and has been for some time. When you have been supported and been able to hit the goals you aimed at in life.

But not everyone has had that experience. And even if they had, there are still times in life when things are not conducive to being positive.

When we are tired or exhausted it is really hard to think positively. There are times when this is very difficult, especially under harsh circumstances or in the middle of major life challenges.

However, there are times when we need to review our lives and risk making a change in our perception, our attitude to something, or our inner self-talk.

To see change as a fearful thing may create resistance, and our thoughts may well echo this.

> **If you keep doing what you've been doing,**
> **You'll keep getting what you've been getting!**

When we recognise that we are having difficulty in this area, we may decide to look at our thoughts in order to find a different mental strategy.

It is little short of insanity to think that if we keep thinking and doing what we have always done, that we will get something different than we have always got.

In other words, if we want different results we need to do or think differently.

Working with Affirmations is becoming quite fashionable. Affirmations are positive statements that are not necessarily true right now, but that we want to focus on in order to manifest them into reality.

What some may not know is that when we try to plant a positive thought into a mind that is chocker-block full of its opposite i.e. - 'I am now rich and prosperous' when you are going through a financial crisis and have poverty issues or fear of being rich – we may find that working with the affirmation may bring up many subconscious beliefs or issues that are contra to the new desired state.

In other words, it can cause aggravation of the condition initially and one may well feel totally overwhelmed by it. This can lead to frustration, failure and prematurely prevent us from continuing through to success.

Finding the right statement for you *at that time* is the key to positive change!

Affirmations - ?

Becoming more aware of where you really are, and working in incremental steps in the direction you want to go will be less stressful. And there is more likelihood of success.

So, find an affirmation that is more realistic to work with, such as 'I am willing to release my fear of having prosperity', 'it is safe to have more money', or 'I am now open to having more money' and gradually 'up' the affirmation statement as you deal with the subconscious reactions to the changes you are instigating.

This in itself is a huge subject, and not to be undertaken lightly. I have spent many years working with and on Affirmations. For it is important to find the correct statements that work directly with you and your issue and the blockage on that issue.

At the very least, ensure that your affirmation is stated in a positive way (don't say 'not' in the wording for instance) that it is believable as a possibility (or the mind will be too busy arguing over it to listen to it) and that it is consistent.

Be aware that creating positive change in your life will take up energy until the change is established. Also be aware that when you start to initiate positive change that you will initially be more tired.

However, the result will pay you back many times over with improved health, efficiency and well-being.

Relax into this as a process. The end is worth it!

Affirmations to Support Health and Healing

If you want to fast rack your health recovery, becoming mindful of any hidden mental or subconscious thoughts that are sabotaging your progress, and working to reverse or remove these will greatly enhance and speed up your successful progress.

You can work them in a variety of ways:

- Work with a kinesiologist to de-stress the statement or affirmation for more efficient change
- Journal your affirmation and inner response in a dedicated manner until there is no more inner argument
- Repeat and nurture the chosen affirmation daily until the fruits of positive change are firmly established
- Dig underneath the statement to the causative factors to create better energy flow in your life and mind

Healing Affirmations

Here are some excellent Affirmations and Statements to de-stress or to use as home-work follow-up. Choose what feels right to you as well as what you aspire to:

1. I am ready to be well, healthy and whole again
2. I recover my health quickly and easily
3. I know what to do to support my recovery
4. It is safe to be in a physical body
5. Despite how I got to this condition, I can re-create a newer and better body and way to be
6. I choose to know myself as a healthy person again
7. My body is fully willing to recover health and energy again
8. My body is easily and fully utilizing all nutritional support for my good health
9. I love my body, and it supports me back
10. I am now healing all disharmony and dis-integration of unity within my body
11. I am open to embracing life and movement again
12. I easily and safely eliminate old and stagnant thoughts and stabilize myself in love
13. I always choose those thoughts that heal, cleanse and support me
14. I always see beauty and love in my body
15. I fully deserve and expect perfect health from now on
16. I easily and lovingly release my pain and disease and allow healing into my heart and body
17. I listen to and honour my body's needs
18. I embrace life and I let go all thoughts of death and dying
19. I choose to heal in all areas of my life

20. I fully accept myself for who I am
21. I deserve to be well and healthy
22. I release the need for having an illness
23. My body is improving itself every day
24. My mind, body, heart and spirit are in perfect balance
25. I am in the process of positive change
26. I learn the underlying lesson and release the testing
27. I exercise in order to enhance my well-being
28. I am friends with my body
29. I am grateful to my body for having served me this far
30. My body belongs to me and to no-one else
31. I take responsibility for my body and for my health
32. I can get well again, and I am now choosing to do so
33. I know when to exert myself, and when to rest
34. I choose to know and experience that life can give me pleasant surprises
35. It is safe to be me

Meditation – Or Not?

Many people the world over find comfort in meditation. It helps them to still the mind, calm the senses, and slow the systems.

There are some people who meditate that I have come into contact with who appear to think that if someone doesn't meditate too, then they are not really 'spiritual' or are not serious about being on their 'path'. Some people judge you according to this, without really checking to see who you are and what works for you – they often think that what works for them or what Swami *Somebodyorother* tells them is the only way to be or act. But there are many roads to Rome or in this case – 'heaven'.

I have become a lot more understanding myself about individual meditation habits and far less judgmental.

Not everyone who doesn't meditate (just like 'them') is a 'lost cause'.

Some are just not built that way, and find their peace with just observing nature, or looking at the stars. Or watching rain drops fall. Or just listening to certain music, or chanting, or anything else that helps them to mentally 'switch gear' and center back again. Or going for a quiet walk to clear their mind...

Friends and clients of mine who have done intensive meditation retreats when not used to it, have sometimes taken months to recover and process the effects of a long meditation intensive. When you have the time and space to fully process and you don't have to hold down a job or career, and don't need to drive in today's traffic, you may find it easier and quicker to complete that type of meditation process.

But we don't all have this luxury.

Taking time out to go 'within' for a week may be sufficient to stir up things for some but please do take care to nurture yourself and allow time to complete the process *afterwards*.

For others, of course, this approach is perfect.

The bottom line is that there are many ways to meditate, and it is important to find your own level of comfort. Don't feel forced into doing something because others think that that is what you 'should' be doing.

If a certain type of meditation works for you, it will certainly help you to free up energy and feel more rejuvenated and also relaxed.

If not, you can try Tai Chi, or Qigong, or Yoga, which when performed properly are all excellent for focus, self development, inner connection and improving energy flow. I know some who paint or even 'color-in' books and this becomes a meditation for them...

Experiment to find out what makes you feel more centered, calm and connected with yourself, rather than what others *tell* you what you should do.

Getting Help

If after reading this book, you recognize something that makes sense to you for your own health-journey and you feel that you could work on a new aspect of your physical, mental or emotional health, please do get some support. In some of the earlier pages there may have been included some suggestions of appropriate assistance that have worked for myself or my clients.

There is a hesitation for me to recommend Hypnotherapists for the Sensitive person, whose boundaries have usually already been compromised. I feel that their goal would be better aimed toward a strengthening of their own boundaries and learning how to refuse access to the mind or energies of others. Having said that, if you are particularly led that way, then it is your choice. I do remember having a session with one hypnotherapist who requested to set up – before I had time to assess and fully realize what he was asking – a trigger password so that he could access my energies at any time... this was intended to be used as a 'coaching' mechanism in order to instruct those hidden aspects of my mind and subconscious whenever necessary. Later I realized that this was not for me due to my own personal history. And instead I focused on healing my boundaries and strengthening from the inside.

I also tend toward a preference toward counseling or psychology rather than Psychiatrists, who tend to prescribe drugs too readily, though in special instances these may help manage symptoms of a depression whilst one works on the underlying causes energetically and emotionally. But please find out what works for you, as I did.

If you prefer to work with a Psychologist or Counselor, please do also consider doing work with an energy therapist or kinesiologist at the same time though not on the same day, obviously. Say see the kinesiologist within one to three days after your counseling session and the issues that have been revealed can be cleared from the energy systems before they get reabsorbed back again. Or you might find it works better for you to alternate sessions so that you are clearing as you are recognizing.

Seeing two practitioners may be a somewhat more expensive initially, but is quicker and more effective in the long run, for that which you uncover in therapy can be cleared out of your body's memory and energy systems more quickly using a combined counseling and energy work approach, which can reduce your need for therapy by many years.

This ultimately means less time in therapy and therefore more time for effective and enjoyable living.

One client who I saw had had many years of counseling and therapy but felt he was still stuck in it all still. After several sessions of energy work he proclaimed that he felt so much better and that he now actually *felt* that he had finally sorted through it all and he also had the benefit of having recognized his issues intellectually. Because he had become aware through therapy of what his issues were, he was now more readily able to recognize that there was a big shift in how he saw things when we cleared the energetic and emotional memories from his energy fields.

To find a good counselor or psychologist, ask about to see who has the kind of manner that makes you feel comfortable. Insist on a brief talk with them to see how they sound, how they feel to you and what they can offer in view of what you would like to work with. It is important to feel you can place some trust in a therapist initially as the work can become intimate.

Kinesiology and other types of therapies and ethical energy work can be very effective, with or without psychology, when you work with someone you feel comfortable with, someone who has training and understanding in the mental as well as emotional areas.

Those who feel more drawn to spiritual healing work, do make sure that your healing therapist has some understanding of the physical and mental state as well as the spiritual and emotional. In other words, work with someone you feel comfortable with, but who is also experienced to take you to the next level.

I do not necessarily discount medical doctors, as they can be magnificent at dealing with those blockages that have become part of our body physiology in the form of disease or illness. They can be masters at surgery. But disease in the body is usually because the energy signals were either not picked up and dealt with, or over time the body has had to deal with too much or has absorbed too much. These are not the only reasons, of course.

The maxim "Prevention is Better than Cure!" will always prevail in my book. For sometimes a roundabout of chemical prescriptions can create further issues or complications, keeping one on a wheel of dependency.

Addressing nutrition is only part of the answer, and I hope that you have discovered far more in these pages.

Fortunately, I have personally come across some medical practitioners who possess a higher degree of awareness regarding natural solutions and therapies and are willing to work side by side with them and you may be lucky to find some that have studied both disciplines.

As we are not just our body, nor just our emotion, nor just our mind or spirit, but a remarkable blend and union of molecules of energy and spirit, we need to address and consider multiple aspects.

If there is *any* health concern, please do get a professional medical opinion.

For your convenience, I have included some ideas for types of therapy support and how they may be able to help you. There are plenty of positive and helpful therapies, these are just some of the more common ones, in case you haven't yet tried them.

HEALING SOLUTIONS

By now you will most certainly be aware, if you weren't already, that healing cannot always be guaranteed if one focuses only on dealing with just the physical symptoms. Though the physical aspect is a very important one, we sometimes need to take steps to deal with other connected aspects. Just as we are social beings and cannot thrive in pure isolation, so too the physical body has many related parts that interact with and are interdependent on each other. True and lasting healing cannot be effected without dealing with more than one component.

The important and major aspects or components of the being that constitutes a functioning human being are:

- Physical
- Emotional
- Mental / Psychological
- Spiritual
- Energetic

Physical

This will include damage sustained in the body. And long (or short) term impact from imbalance or suffering from any of the other components of the being. It will also include symptoms of nervous system issues whether from an emotional, spiritual, energetic or mental cause.

Emotional

Emotions can be influenced by any of the other being's constituents, and a sustained problem in this area can result in a habitual hormonal imbalance with the consequential residual toxicity in the body. So dealing with physical toxicity, whilst addressing and resetting the hormonal balance as well as addressing underlying emotional responses or past hurt and damage (on an emotional and mental level) can begin to make vast improvement to the being's ability to cope with everyday emotional issues naturally as well as to prevent collapse from further highly charged emotional moments.

Mental / Psychological

Self talk is often blamed for mental issues, but the impact of past negative talk from care-givers or those we valued highly whilst in a vulnerable position also cannot be ignored. Bullying, violence and abuse leave their mark, and can dint the mental and emotional resilience of many, so nurturing and supporting a healthy self esteem whilst dealing with repairing past damage and its subsequent physical impact and fall-out that has led to a compromised self image will help to create a new and stronger sense of self.

Recognition of one's internal talk, no matter where the talk was seeded or recorded from, and re-educating the mind to what supports one's mental health and resilience will prevent further mind collapse.

Spiritual

Each of us has an inner self, and one which we are not always in touch with. From this self comes our self expression and moral compass, which is separate from the expression of our personality and does not depend on others for approval. Our inner compass reflects the quality of our spirit, as not all spirits are equal. Having a meaningful spiritual life can be essential to the sensitive type of person, as it enables them to make sense of the world they find themselves in. The harshness of some experiences can compromise and bruise the spirit, and this can depress the immune system. So recovering one's spiritual mojo or healing any spiritual abuse or damage can be an important step when this aspect figures in the original cause of ill health.

Energetic

Energy is not just about fuel for the body, nor what is expended by the body. Energy is what we run on, it is the base unit of the fire and spark within us, which can erupt with a pure joy even when one is totally exhausted, but can also down us like a brick even when it would appear to others that we have just won our biggest victory. Our spirit is a truly remarkable aspect, and is the very soul beyond our mind, the very heart beyond our head and reasoning, and has great impact on our energetic "tone" and function.

The energetic aspect also covers the energy systems within the body, and these manage the overall functioning of the body through its various physical processes. These energy systems reach into the physical but meld both spiritual, mental, emotional and physical together.

A blockage in the energetic system such as a meridian (discovered and developed by the ancient Chinese) can compromise function of an organ, gland or complete physical system, and has the power to affect the associated related emotional tone.

So including this aspect when addressing one's healing process can more efficiently marry all aspects of the being toward good health again.

Using nature and the 13 Basic Health Factors will support any energy work that you do.

Another component to healing energetically is to work energetically, and this can include energy healing work, TCM, acupuncture, tai chi and affirmations.

Affirmations can be very powerful when combined with other forms of healing and support, as it can help deal with the causal factors underlying an imbalance. Being aware of what we feed our mind, our thoughts, our hearts and of how these affect our body and its functioning, and using Affirmations to embed new thoughts and ways of thinking can be an extremely powerful tool!

Healing The Whole

Health is not just a physical thing, though that is where ill-health symptoms show the most obviously – health is the correct functioning of all of the various components of the being, a harmony with heart and mind and body and spirit.

Finding what works for you and what is appropriate, be it counselor and osteopath, or kinesiologist and acupuncture or psychologist and affirmations, or any other combinations that feel right for you, will exponentially enhance your healing process. For you are addressing more than just the body or just the mind.

Therapy Solutions:

OSTEOPATHY, PHYSIOTHERAPY, BOWEN THERAPY, CHIROPRACTIC, ELECTRO-ACUPUNCTURE, FELDENKRAIS,

All of the above therapies assist the physical body initially. They can align the skeleton, support the Nervous System, help to release frozen trauma through accidents, operations or illness held still in the body, as well as reset tendons, ligaments and muscles. Some therapists are also trained in kinesiology, which is a real enhancement to their diagnostic and support abilities.

All physical therapies will have impact on all of the other aspects of the being, though the effect and benefit will often depend on how the initial imbalance in health came about. So a combination of therapies that approach and deal with all of the aspects more directly in some way will be of the greatest effect and efficiency.

KINESIOLOGY

This can be a valuable tool, as it can help to expose hidden stresses, stressors, and issues. It is often combined with body work when the kinesiologist links it with acupressure massage or physical movements and exercises. It can also be used with vibrational supports or energy medicines, such as flower or gem essences or homeopathic medicines. Because it works on several levels, it can be quite impactful.

NATUROPATHY, HOMEOPATHY, HERBS

These therapies work on providing the right nutritional food supplement or oral medicine to not only support the body, but also to assist in bringing in positive change.

MASSAGE

This serves to promote circulation, and to clear toxicity caught in the cells. It is also a feel-good reward that can help to relax the body and to slow the mind. It is a positive adjunct to energy work or in between visits to the chiropractor or osteopath.

TCM – Traditional Chinese Medicine

TCM practitioners often combine herbs, acupuncture, acupressure massage, shiatsu and cupping to achieve balance in the body. Primarily focusing on the meridians and tone of the pulse, they can help to detoxify the body, clear energy channels, improve body and emotion function and strengthen one's vitality.

YOGA, TAI CHI, MEDITATION

Some of these are self-doable once you know how. They can assist in centering the mind, bringing balance back into the emotions and physical body again, as well as being positive stress managers. They can also be used to bring deeper introspection and the space to move through deep issues if you choose.

NUTRITION

Filtered water, Organic products, non GMO foods, foods in season, appropriate nutritional supplementation to replace deficiencies, herbs for health, avoiding toxic ingredients both in the body and on the body will all support your health recovery.

WHERE TO NEXT?

We have looked at some of the reasons for tiredness and lack of energy. We have examined some ideas relating to the physical body, emotion, and the energy bodies, as well as possible blocks to health.

We have considered some hidden reasons and attitudes that can prevent good health and inner peace. We have also uncovered some important reasons why we may not be as healthy as we could be, and what we can do about them.

Health and Energy is more than just treating the physical body. It is more than just exercise, massage, or taking the right Super-foods.

Energetic impacts can often compromise health. One truth is that when undergoing any kind of change, the body itself may well need increased support in order to hold the new understanding and consciousness.

If the body is not strong enough or is not supported, it may well find it hard to contain and maintain a positive shift in energy, and may tend to collapse, so to speak, back on itself, ending up feeling the same old way and doing the same old thing. With little final gain.

Healing needs to take place on several levels together.

Understanding how hidden issues can affect the efficiency of any given healing protocol or regime, whether chemical, nutritional or energetic can greatly assist in providing optimum results for your efforts.

We need to understand the power of our own thoughts and words, and to use them for our benefit. We need to recognise those blockages still preventing the longed for improvement in our health, such as hidden toxicity or lack of mineral support and even more simply, the basic elements that are required for health.

We also need to associate with healing frequencies, as well as to uncover any hidden reasons *not* to change. Knowing that mercury toxicity can be found in things we have taken for granted and what its effects are on the nervous system, as well as how to clear it from the system can give us further insight into improving our health and vitality.

We are all being called to take responsibility for our own health, and not to rely solely on the doctor, as nutrition cannot be found in a tablet, nor ultimate knowledge in a medical catalogue.

Health is one of our biggest assets. When we have our health, we have the capability to do so much, to achieve so much and to function in a way that does not leave us dependent on others.

Regaining health is about treating the whole person. About looking at the whole of life.

And sometimes it is necessary to deal with the past (or sometimes the future) in order to manage the present.

When we get the positive spin, the lesson or gift if you like, on our experiences, we can move on.

I wish you well on your search for full health, energy and life.

Good Health,

Myra Sri

FURTHER INFORMATION

References for this book:

Some reference links to confirm the above:

Mercury:

- http://articles.mercola.com/sites/articles/archive/2013/02/05/mercury-un-treaty-abolishes-amalgam.aspx
- http://www.fda.gov/downloads/Adviso...e/DentalProductsPanel/UCM236379.pdf
- http://www.government.se/sb/d/11459/a/118550

Minerals:

- http://www.sciences360.com/index.php/minerals-needed-for-healthy-growth-656/
- www.mercola.com - Zinc

Vaccinations:

- http://www.collective-evolution.com/2014/01/28/you-want-to-vaccinate-my-child-no-problem-just-sign-this-form/
- http://www.naturalnews.com/048430_vaccines_sudden_death_big_pharma.html#ixzz3qc2rlnpg
- https://www.youtube.com/watch?v=1VqydXmBBFs - BILL GATES – GMO Depopulation
- https://www.youtube.com/watch?v=7XRUEuVP2qE - BILL GATES Depopulation

Inflammation:

- http://livingbyheart.tripod.com/sitebuildercontent/sitebuilderfiles/timearticlesecretkiller.pdf
- http://abcnews.go.com/Health/WellnessNews/story?id=8450036 Milk

- omega-3 and omega-6 fats needs to be in balance
- http://theconsciouslife.com/omega-3-6-9-ratio-cooking-oils.htm
- http://abcnews.go.com/Health/WellnessNews/story?id=8450036
- http://theconsciouslife.com/top-10-inflammatory-foods-to-avoid.htm
- http://www.care2.com/greenliving/top-12-foods-that-cause-inflammation.html

"Acupuncture and the Chakra Energy System" John R Cross

Other products you may be interested in:

Energy Secrets Series – Books

Secrets Beyond Aromatherapy

Secrets Behind Energy Fields

New Crystal Codes – Align to the New Energies

Secrets to Serene Space – Space Clearing

Guided Meditations at www.myrasri.com/new-healing-store

The New Evolved Chakras – Chakra Alignment

The Highly Sensitive's Guide to the Sensory Psychic Chakras

BOOKS DUE FOR PUBLICATION SOON:

Affirmations; - I intend to also write about Affirmations and the best ways of using and working with them. Stay tuned to my website www.myrasri.com or register your interest by signing up for my newsletter.

FREE NEWSLETTER:

Get my free newsletter which lets you know when there are special deals and offers, new meditations and books, as well as current news items on life, challenge, change, self help healing, self empowerment and spirituality.

Sign up obligation-free here: www.myrasri.com

About the Author

Myra Sri was born in England and later moved to Australia in her twenties with her then husband and two young children. As an Indigo-Sensitive person, she always maintained a spiritual leaning.

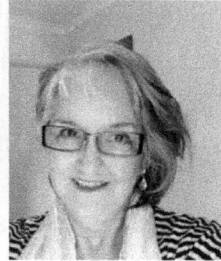

Life and health issues challenged her naivety in blind religious faith. Myra embarked on the reconstruction of her life and the discovery of her true identity.

Through her journeying and in questing for solutions to her own compromised health, she discovered complementary and natural therapies. Undertaking extensive training and study she became an energy healing practitioner and kinesiologist. Qualifying as an instructor in several modalities, she subsequently discovered where there was a lack of teaching and understanding and set upon further research and discovery, resulting in her own unique advanced workshops which have been taught around Australia since the early 1990's. These continuing experiences led her to develop her own innate skills and supported her in re-member-ing her healing skills and psychic abilities.

Running her own private practice since the late 80's, Myra remains an avid explorer and student of evolving ways to heal and support the soul and spirit.

She wrote her first book together with doctors and a group of other professionals in 2006. Discoveries since 2001 of the newly evolving Chakra systems were diarised and documented. After further research, then developing and teaching courses on these, Myra was invited to teach in England and Germany in 2011. Freshly inspired to further document her discoveries, Myra returned to Australia to write about the current energy shifts since the turn of the millennium. Further books were authored on how these energies were affecting essential oils and crystal energies. The Energy Healing Secrets Series is presented to assist in self help, self healing and growth toward spiritual mastery.

The book on New Evolved Chakras is based on the *New Evolved Chakras Workshop series* which includes the new Earthing Chakras, the Psychic Body Chakras and the Signal-Survival Chakras. The discovery of these extraordinary Chakras have also been confirmed by other spiritual teachers and psychics to be instrumental in everybody's healing process and the book on these Chakras is soon to be published.

Myra provides a safe and attentive healing space for her clients and students, and works multi-dimensionally, enabling major energy and spiritual shifts. Her focus is on the Soul and spirit. Considered a resort for difficult or complicated situations, she has often been referred to as 'the Healer's Healer'.

Myra works multi-dimensionally, enabling major energy and spiritual shifts.

WORKSHOPS:

Some of Myra's workshops include:

Past Life Training – Navigating Soul Journey and Genetic Issues and Karma safely

HygienEthics Series (Protection and Energy Management Series) – Working With Energy, Living With Energy, Being Energy, Protection HygienEthics, HygienEthics for Therapists, Advanced HygienEthics

Navigating Life – Mastery Journey Series

Muscle Testing Basics

Crystal Workshops

New Evolved Chakra Series - New Earthing Chakras, New Psychic Body and Chakras, New Signal-Survival Chakras

SECRETS Beyond Aromatherapy

CHAKRA HEALING SECRETS
ETHERIC COLOUR CODES
TRANSFORMATION SECRETS

Behind the Invisible Etheric Codes
of Essential Oils
Chakra and Energy Healing Secrets
for the New Era

MYRA SRI

Secrets Behind Energy Fields

BECOME YOUR OWN ENERGY GURU
RECLAIM YOUR ENERGY & VITALITY

MYRA SRI

SECRETS to SERENE SPACE

SPACE CLEARING
ATIVE ENERGIES
PHYSICS AND
IS TO CHANGE
E AND LIFE

Secret TRUTHS Health & Well-Being

HEALTH TRUTHS THAT EVERYONE SHOULD KNOW
TOXICITY AND THE NERVOUS SYSTEM
SECRETS BEYOND NUTRITION

Resolve Exhaustion and Tiredness NATURALLY!
Recognise Obstacles to Health and Vitality
Body-Mind and Emotion to Hook

MYRA SRI

The NEW CRYSTAL CODES

Align Your Crystals To The New Energies

CRYSTAL CODES, CIPHERS AND FUNCTIONS
FOR THE NEW BRA
New: ALIGN YOUR CRYSTALS
CHOOSING AND WORKING WITH CRYSTALS

Learn the difference between crystals
Sets of crystals to attract more love, success, protection, life stress

MYRA SRI

The beauty and power of Essential Oils has been known to us for thousands of years, from Ancient Indian healers to current day aromatherapists.

Few were aware of etheric Colour Codes of Essential Oils.

Until now!

Essential Oils, like the Chakra systems, have evolved and Come of Age.

Their abilities have expanded and they are now poised ready to assist us all as we work with and move fully into the new energies of this new Era.

Come on a journey into the astounding colours of oils; see how they interact with human senses and subtle body anatomy. Learn their impacts and the unseen implications with the Soul and incarnational aspects. Discover which Chakras respond best, and which energy system is most enhanced by their actions. You may be pleasantly surprised!

The basic etheric body colours of the human energy systems appeared to have undergone change. Even the Main Chakras are responding differently to colour and vibration. It would seem that no longer do most of us reflect (and often poorly at that) the basic opaque paint-box-type colours previously associated with the seven basic colours of the rainbow – some of us are now able to reflect more glorious and colourful hues and iridescences from and through the auric layers and chakras when balanced correctly.

Living in cities can prevent some of these new hues and their tints from shining within and without, as the electromagnetic smog and pollution can lower the frequencies to a paler and poorer version. In these times it is becoming more important to reconnect back to nature, the land or the sea, purer energies, higher vibrations and natural remedies whenever and wherever possible to sustain us. And the essential oils are part of this remedy.

The humble oil along with knowledge of its inherent etheric colour codes and abilities will further enhance everyone's experience of the nature and the knowing that is held within each loving oil and hidden within the etheric world itself, and will further enhance and amplify all of your current benefits when used with the increased awareness.

Recognize the New Roles that these amazing gifts from our Planet are playing right now.

Explore the Etheric Colours of over Thirty Essential Oils. Learn their Secrets.

Find new and powerful ways of working with them.

Spend time with them. Let your choice of Oil reveal to you further hidden information to assist you with your client or with your own personal transformation.

Work with Essential Oils in ways you've never done before!

Amazon Reviews:

A treasure of energetic information

Thrilled with the content of this book and I have read almost every aromatherapy book there is

I wonder why this book is not used as a textbook

When we have good health, we really do have a huge asset at the ready – there is no price to be placed on it as from our good health so many positive things can arise. When we are exhausted and tired through dealing with other peoples issues, emotions and energies, we are cheating ourselves of our true destiny and life journey.

Nobody lives as an entire isolated and energetic island to themselves. We are all social beings and part of life is social interaction of some kind or another. Which also means energetic interaction - the contact that takes place on those unseen levels, yet we can still feel their action and their impact.

When we don't know where our energy goes, when we work with others closely, when we are faced with emotional or traumatic scenes, when others think it is ok and acceptable to explode around us, when we think there must be something wrong with us because of what we continually encounter in our life, we need answers to what is happening, and what we can do about it!

Learning to navigate through life in energies that are less than positive or harmonious sometimes requires outside information or help. And all you really need to invest is some of your time and energy to become your own energy guru and healer.

Here is a collection of techniques, exercises and tools that are proven energy strengtheners. Selected from the many workshops I have taught on this topic are easy, effective solutions and understandings for anybody who is involved with other people and not coping as well as they could.

You can begin to reclaim your own identity and autonomy again, and easily recognise who and what has been affecting you with the easy to follow instructions and ideas.

Be successful and happy, protect your energy and let good health and good energy be your positive foundation.

A new look at the Art of Space Clearing. Clear Negative Energies and Use Metaphysics to Change Your Space and Life. Become your own Guru. Learn the Art of Creating Sanctuary, within and without...

A home is a place to return to for safety, nurturing, rejuvenation and love. Does your home sanctuary nurture and support you? Does it fill you with pleasure and enjoyment?

Take a moment to look around your home... how does it reflect you? How does it feel to you? Are you able to revitalise and rejuvenate there whenever you need to? Does your home welcome you? If the answer is "No" and you are aware that you need to do something to change your space, and possibly yourself, then you will find lots of ideas and help in this book.

If you want to go deeper than just shifting surface stuff around, if you feel that there could be some old "nasties" lying around somewhere that you would like to shift, if you feel that you would like to get clearer within yourself as well as within your living space, then this is the book for you!

Decluttering may be needed. Or it could be that there are some old or negative energies to clear. What about the sense of being "spied" on? Learn about how to remove not only "nasties" but also learn what a Portal is and how to clear these, as well as Orbs and Thoughtforms. Discover not only how to Clear your place and enhance your home and life, but the crucial and essential step that must follow for true and lasting success in your Clearing.

Here in an easy to read book you will find how to create Sanctuary in your own personal space with time-proven tools. Decluttering is made easy. Imprints are explained and removal instructions are included together with further powerful techniques to incorporate into your ritual or chosen exercise to bring healing into the home. This is a true self help book!

Since the huge energy shifts of recent years, frequencies have been updated in many areas. The discovery of the new Evolved Chakras has demonstrated that we are all in a process of upgrade and re-alignment. This includes not only the human subtle bodies but also the energetic frequencies of oils and crystals.

This book contains clear instructions on How to Align your Evolved Crystal to the New Incoming Energies.

The author shares her knowledge on the new Crystal Codes and Ciphers, as well as how to read where your crystals energies are at and how to align them with the new Era frequencies.

You will not find this knowledge anywhere else. This little book also has everything you need to identify the different functions and powers of Quartz Crystals and much, much more.

You will learn about how to connect to your crystal, how to care for it, code and program it and how to use it wisely. You will find in these pages ideas that will inspire you to love and journey with your chosen gem.

You will also learn how to identify various types of crystals, some metaphysical properties, sets of crystals and learn the difference between an Isis crystal, a Record-Keeper, a Lemurian and much more...

Make the most of your willing crystal and harness its energies for the new energy shifts right now!

This is cutting edge information and the time is ripe to re-energise your crystal.